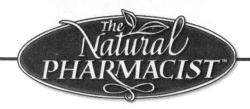

The Natural PHARMACIST™

Inside—Find the Answers to These Questions and More

☑ How well does St. John's wort work for depression? (See page 71.)

☑ How much should I take? (See page 86.)

☑ What kind of St. John's wort should I take? (See page 86.)

☑ Are there any side effects? (See page 106.)

☑ Does St. John's wort interact with any medications? (See page 110.)

☑ Is there anyone who should *not* take St. John's wort? (See page 99.)

☑ How long does it take before I start seeing results? (See page 87.)

☑ What are the other natural treatments I can use for depression? (See page 141.)

☑ I have anxiety with my depression, what are my options? (See page 155.)

☑ I have insomnia with my depression, what are my options? (See page 158.)

☑ How does St. John's wort compare to prescription drugs? (See page 115.)

W9-ACA-201

THE NATURAL PHARMACIST Library

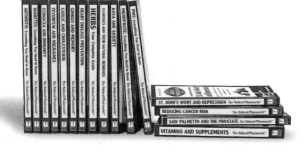

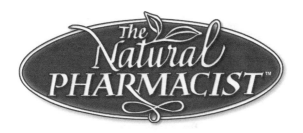

Everything You Need to Know About

St. John's Wort and Depression

Steven Bratman, M.D.

Series Editors

Steven Bratman, M.D.

David Kroll, Ph.D.

A DIVISION OF PRIMA PUBLISHING

Visit us online at www.thenaturalpharmacist.com

Warning—Disclaimer

This book is not intended to provide medical advice and is sold with the understanding that the publisher and the author are not liable for the misconception or misuse of information provided. The author and Prima Publishing shall have neither liability nor responsibility to any person or entity with respect to any loss, damage, or injury caused or alleged to be caused directly or indirectly by the information contained in this book or the use of any products mentioned. Readers should not use any of the products discussed in this book without the advice of a medical professional.

The Food and Drug Administration has not approved the use of any of the natural treatments discussed in this book. This book, and the information contained herein, has not been approved by the Food and Drug Administration.

Pseudonyms are used throughout to protect the privacy of individuals involved.

PRIMA HEALTH and colophon are trademarks of Prima Communications, Inc.

THE NATURAL PHARMACIST™ is a trademark of Prima Communications, Inc.

Illustrations by Helene D. Stevens. Illustrations © 1999 Prima Publishing. All rights reserved.

All products mentioned in this book are trademarks of their respective companies.

Library of Congress Cataloging-in-Publication Data

Bratman, Steven.
    St. John's wort and depression / Steven Bratman.
        p.   cm.—(The natural pharmacist)
    Includes bibliographical references and index.
    ISBN 0-7615-1553-4
    1. Depression, Mental—Alternative treatment.   2. Triadenum virginicum—
Therapeutic use.
    3. Herbs—Therapeutic use.   I. Title.   II. Series.
    RC537.B7473 1999
    616.85'2706—dc21   98-17492
                                                                            CIP

                99 00 01 02 HH 10 9 8 7 6 5 4 3 2 1
                    Printed in the United States of America

Visit us online at www.thenaturalpharmacist.com

Contents

What Makes This Book Different?

The interest in natural medicine has never been greater. According to the National Association of Chain Drug Stores, 65 million Americans are using natural supplements, and the number is growing! Yet, it is hard for the consumer to find trustworthy sources for balanced information about this emerging field. Why? Frankly, natural medicine has had a checkered history. From snake oil potions sold at the turn of the century to those books, magazines, and product catalogs that hype miracle cures today, this is a field where exaggerated claims have been the norm. Proponents of natural medicine have tended to abuse science, treating it more as a marketing tool than a means of discovering the truth.

But there is truth to be found. Studies of vitamins, minerals, and other food supplements have been with us since these nutritional substances were first discovered, and the level and quality of this science has grown dramatically in the last 20 years. Herbal medicine has been neglected in the United States, but in Europe, this, the oldest of all healing arts, has been the subject of tremendous and ongoing scientific interest.

At present, for a number of herbs and supplements, it is possible to give reasonably scientific answers to the questions: How well does this work? How safe is it? What types of conditions is it best used for?

THE NATURAL PHARMACIST series is designed to cut through the hype and tell you what we know and what we don't know about popular natural treatments. These books are more conservative than any others available, more honest about the weaknesses of natural approaches, more fair in their comparisons of natural and conventional treatments. You won't find any miracle cures here, but you will discover useful options that can help you become healthier.

Why Choose Natural Treatments?

Although the science behind natural medicine continues to grow, this is still a much less scientifically validated field than conventional medicine. You might ask, "Why should I resort to an herb that is only partly proven, when I could take a drug with solid science behind it?" There are at least three good reasons to consider natural alternatives.

First, some herbs and supplements offer benefits that are not matched by any conventional drug. Vitamin E is a good example. It appears to help prevent prostate cancer, a benefit that no standard medication can claim. Also, vitamin E almost certainly helps prevent heart disease. While there are standard drugs that also prevent heart disease, vitamin E works differently and may be able to complement many of the other approaches.

Another example is the herb milk thistle. Studies strongly suggest that this herb can protect the liver from injury. There is no pill or tablet your doctor can prescribe to do the same.

Even if the science behind some of these treatments is less than perfect, when the risks are low and the possible benefit high, a natural treatment may be worth trying. It is a little-known fact that for many conventional treatments the science is less than perfect as well, and physicians must balance uncertain benefits against incompletely understood risks.

A second reason to consider natural therapies is that some may offer benefits comparable to those of drugs with fewer side effects. The herb St. John's wort is a good example. Reasonably strong scientific evidence suggests that this herb is an effective treatment for mild to moderate depression, while producing fewer side effects on average than conventional medications. Saw palmetto for benign enlargement of the prostate, ginkgo for relieving symptoms and perhaps slowing the progression of Alzheimer's disease, and glucosamine for osteoarthritis are other examples. This is not to say that herbs and supplements are completely harmless—they're not—but for most the level of risk is quite low.

Finally, there is a philosophical point to consider. For many people, it "feels" better to use a treatment that comes from nature instead of from a laboratory. Just as you might rather wear all-cotton clothing than polyester, or look at a mountain landscape rather than the skyscrapers of a downtown city, natural treatments may simply feel more compatible with your view of life. We can quibble endlessly about just what "natural" means and whether a certain treatment is "actually" natural or not, but such arguments are beside the point. The difference is in the feeling, and feelings matter. In fact, having a good feeling about taking an herb may lead you to use it more consistently than you would a prescription drug.

Of course, at times synthetic drugs may be necessary and even lifesaving. But on many other occasions it may be quite reasonable to turn to an herb or supplement instead of a drug.

To make good decisions you need good information. Unfortunately, while hundreds of books on alternative medicine are published every year, many are highly misleading. The phrase "studies prove" is often used when the studies in question are so small or so badly conducted that they prove nothing at all. You may even find that the "data" from other books comes from studies with petri dishes and not real people!

You can't even assume that books written by well-known authors are scientifically sound. Many of these authors rely on secondary writers, leading to a game of "telephone," where misconceptions are passed around from book to book. And there's a strong tendency to exaggerate the power of natural remedies, whitewashing them with selective reporting.

THE NATURAL PHARMACIST series gives you the balanced information you need to make informed decisions about your health needs. Setting a new, high standard of accuracy and objectivity, these books take a realistic look at the herbs and supplements you read about in the news. You will encounter both favorable and unfavorable studies in these pages and will learn about both the benefits and the risks of natural treatments.

THE NATURAL PHARMACIST series is the source you can trust.

Steven Bratman, M.D.
David Kroll, Ph.D.

Introduction

Every year, millions of people seek treatment for depression, complaining of symptoms that interfere with their relationships, impair their work capacity, and deprive them of the full emotional experiences of life. For most of this century, psychotherapy has been the primary treatment for mild to moderate depression. However, psychotherapy is slow, expensive, and not always entirely successful. Many people complain that they continue to experience depression even after years of otherwise useful psychotherapy.

Treatment for depression was revolutionized in the late 1980s with the production of Prozac, the first antidepressant drug truly appropriate for mild to moderate depression. Breaking all previous records for the use of antidepressants, Prozac quickly achieved what can only be described as cult status. "Tess," a woman made famous in Peter Kramer's *Listening to Prozac,* called herself "Ms. Prozac" because she believed the drug gave her "charisma, courage, character, and social competency." So positive was Prozac's image for a time, it was widely called vitamin P.

Then a backlash set in: Prozac was found to be not nearly so side-effect–free as initially hoped. Real-life experiences revealed that Prozac (and similar drugs) sometimes caused unpleasant symptoms ranging from merely annoying to absolutely intolerable.

Some individuals on Prozac develop insomnia so severe that they must take a second drug at night to sleep. Women frequently complain of decreased libido and the inability to experience orgasm. Other common problems include anxiety, agitation, severe headaches, undesired weight loss, tremors, sweating, and short-term memory loss.

Interestingly, at the same time as the United States was embracing Prozac, a completely different course was taken in Germany. Instead of turning to a new prescription drug, physicians there rediscovered an ancient treatment: the herb St. John's wort. Today, only 7% of the antidepressant prescriptions in Germany are written for Prozac; St. John's wort dominates the field.

Yet, St. John's wort was almost unknown in the United States until quite recently. This situation suddenly changed in early 1997, when strongly positive reporting in *Newsweek* and *The Washington Post,* and on *USA Weekend* and *20/20,* catapulted St. John's wort into public awareness. In successive months, St. John's wort became one of the best-selling herbs in U.S. history.

Nonetheless, St. John's wort is not a panacea. It has its strengths and weaknesses like all other medical treatments, and the research evidence for its effectiveness needs to be strengthened. But for individuals who seek help for symptoms of mild to moderate depression and want a gentler, more natural approach than drugs, St. John's wort could indeed be a splendid option. This book will fairly examine the evidence, to help you decide whether this herb might be useful for you.

What Is
St. John's Wort?

Known officially as *Hypericum perforatum,* St. John's wort is a perennial herb with many branches and bright yellow flowers. It is fond of sun-exposed slopes and grows in dry grasslands, pastures, and sparse woods and alongside roadways. For its beautiful golden petals, St. John's wort is one of the most admired wild plants in Germany, but a more subtle artistic effect can be discovered on close inspection of the leaves. When held up to the light, a kind of watermark can be seen: translucent dots scattered in a pleasing pattern. It is these visual "perforations" that give it the species name *perforatum* (see figure 1).

Another distinguishing characteristic is the numerous black dots on the sepals and petals of the flower. These release a red pigment when squeezed: the "blood" of Saint John, according to tradition.

Like all medicinal herbs, St. John's wort is a weed; in this case a powerful one. When it was brought over to the Americas by Europeans, *Hypericum* became an invasive pest in the Pacific Northwest. It invaded pastures

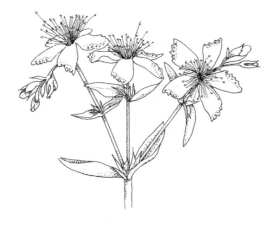

Figure 1. *St. John's wort*

and ranchland in the Klamath area and threatened to become the kudzu of the north. Because cattle that devour large quantities of the herb can develop severe sunburn, local ranchers gave it the epithet "Klamath weed" and undertook to stamp it out with poisons.

Herbicides, however, failed to make an impact. In 1946 *Chrysolina quadregemina Rossi,* an Australian beetle that possessed a voracious appetite for the herb, was introduced as a kind of biological control. (Perhaps the beetles suffered from chronic depression.) *This* intervention was successful, and within 10 years wild St. John's wort was reduced to 1% of its previous prevalence in Northern California. Ironically, these beetles may become a significant obstacle to the intentional U.S. cultivation of St. John's wort now underway.

Why Is It Called St. John's Wort?

Wort is simply an Old English word for a plant or an herb. There are many explanations for the traditional connection to Saint John, but perhaps the simplest is that the herb flowers around the time of the feast of Saint John. Also, in Christian tradition, Saint John represents spiritual light coming to earth. The bright yellow color of the flowers may have thus clinched the connection by seeming to represent fragments of the sun brought close to the ground.

It is tempting to speculate further that antidepressant effects of this herb may have provided another connection with Saint John. Spiritual light is the antithesis of depression. If you feel depressed, you might say that you feel "plunged into darkness"; and when you recover your friends might say that you've "brightened up." Even advertisements for antidepressant drugs make use of this connection by, for example, showing a patient rising from bed and opening a brightly lit window.

Wort **is simply an Old English word for a plant or an herb.**

Those who take St. John's wort often report that they feel a sensation like increased interior light. In the devout environment of the Middle Ages, this experience might well have been interpreted as the presence of a light-bearing saint.

The genus name *Hypericum* also has a meaningful history. According to the noted herbalist Christopher Hobbs, an older name for the genus was *Hyperikon,* deriving from the combination of the words *hyper* (above) and *eikon* (a figure with supernatural characteristics). Hobbs relates this derivation to the traditional use of St. John's wort as a protection against demons, witches, and other supernatural beings. Because our ancestors attributed symptoms of depression to the influence of demonic forces, could it be that the name *Hypericum* indicates that St. John's wort relieved symptoms of depression?

What Is in St. John's Wort?

If the crushed flowers of St. John's wort are steeped in vegetable oil for several weeks, the liquid takes on deep red tones that fluoresce in sunlight. The fluorescent constituent is a chemical named *hypericin*. While this substance is commonly cited as the herb's active ingredient, this has not been proven, and most experts do not believe that hypericin itself is an effective antidepressant. Like all herbs, St. John's wort contains innumerable organic chemicals in varying concentrations. It's most likely that another ingredient, or combination of ingredients, is actually responsible for the antidepressant effect. Hyperforin, for instance, has recently been proposed as the active ingredient, but this too has not been proven.

Because our ancestors attributed symptoms of depression to the influence of demonic forces, could it be that the name *Hypericum* indicates that St. John's wort relieved symptoms of depression?

An abbreviated list of the constituents of St. John's wort includes the species-specific naphthodianthrones hypericin, pseudohypericin, protohypericin, protopseudohypericin, cyclopseudohypericin, and hyperforin as well as nonspecies-specific phenylpropanes, flavonol glycosides, biflavones, tannins and proanthocyanidins, and volatile oils. More on what is known about the chemical basis of St. John's wort's mood-elevating properties is discussed in chapter 5.

What Was St. John's Wort Used for Historically?

From the times of the ancient Greeks, plants of the genus *Hypericum* have been used for a variety of medicinal purposes, such as healing burns and other skin injuries, counteracting snake bites, treating ulcers, and improving the flow of urine. St. John's wort was used in Celtic religious practices in England, and subsequently the herb took on an unofficial spiritual significance among Christians. European herbalists frequently called it *Fuga daemonum,* in reference to the widespread belief that St. John's wort could drive away demons. Thus again we return to the spiritual connotations of St. John's wort.

Perhaps the attribution of supernatural powers to St. John's wort was an archaic response to antidepressant effects. If you lived in Europe in the Middle Ages and your neighbor was unaccountably sad, troubled by guilt, and crippled by anxiety, you would very likely come to believe that he or she was afflicted by demons. If your neighbor then started to drink a daily brew of St. John's wort tea and subsequently recovered from this "demonic possession," you probably couldn't fail to assign magical potency to the herb. It would not be very long before you might feel inspired to use the herb as a symbolic protection, perhaps by wearing it about your neck. An old poem shows this reverence clearly:

> *St. John's Wort doth charm all the witches away,*
> *If gathered at midnight on the saint's holy day.*
> *And devils and witches have no power to harm*
> *Those that do gather the plant for a charm.*

If we in modern times were similarly inclined, I could easily imagine people wearing a necklace of Prozac pills to ward off gloomy thoughts. While I have never heard of anyone taking quite that course, it is not at all unusual for

Prozac Fashion

Actually, Prozac necklaces may not be so far-fetched. There have been recent news reports of jewelry fashioned to look like Prozac and other drugs. Although meant merely as an offbeat fashion statement, such jewelry could actually produce a positive subconscious effect.

people on Prozac to use the drug as a kind of mental amulet. Whenever they suffer rejection or another experience likely to provoke depression, they remind themselves that they are "under the protection of Prozac" and needn't fear emotional collapse. This positive self-suggestion is quite sensible, but it amounts to a talismanic use of the drug. In this respect we are no different from our medieval ancestors who felt reassured by the presence of St. John's wort, whether internally or externally.

St. John's Wort's Entry into Modern Medicine

When scientific medicine began to predominate, references to the psychological effects of St. John's wort started to take a more modern turn. Literature from the early nineteenth century suggested the use of St. John's wort for mood disorders. The first quasi-scientific study on St. John's wort was published in 1939.[1]

In recent decades the development of chemical antidepressants has inspired European scientists to look for similar properties in St. John's wort. Early studies focused on determining whether the constituents of St. John's wort functioned similarly to a class of antidepressants known as

MAO inhibitors (see chapter 4). Later research focused on a serotonin connection (see chapter 5). At the same time, formal trials were begun to determine the clinical effectiveness of St. John's wort in the treatment of depression. The results were so positive that by 1988 St. John's wort was officially approved as an antidepressant drug in Germany.

During the period of explosive growth of Prozac use in the United States, St. John's wort became the dominant antidepressant treatment in Germany and was soon widely used in other European countries as well. In 1993, the latest year for which records are available, German physicians issued more than 2.7 million prescriptions for St. John's wort.

The culture of conventional medicine in Europe is rather receptive to herbal treatment. In the United States, however, herbs have long fallen out of favor in conventional medical practice. But in 1996 the prestigious *British Journal of Medicine* published a review article generally favorable to St. John's wort. This soon caught the attention of the American news media, launching a tidal wave of interest. St. John's wort started to fly off health-food store shelves in quantities never before seen, and major pharmacy chains began to offer it. Doctors, psychologists, and psychotherapists have started to recommend St. John's wort

Former trials were begun to determine the clinical effectiveness of St. John's wort in the treatment of depression. The results were so positive that by 1988 St. John's wort was officially approved as an antidepressant drug in Germany.

to their patients, and the National Institutes of Health (NIH) has launched a major study that will compare this herb against the standard antidepressant drug Zoloft. Never in modern times has an herb made such an impact in the United States.

Unlike some other alternative treatments, St. John's wort actually has enough research behind it to deserve this attention. But before discussing the evidence regarding its use for depression, I must first interpose a brief discussion of depression itself.

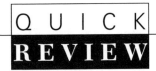

QUICK REVIEW

- St. John's wort has been used as medicine since ancient Greek times.
- Although the concept of depression is a modern one, many of the ancient uses of St. John's wort may have helped treat depression.
- The results of German scientific research suggests that St. John's wort is indeed an effective antidepressant treatment.
- St. John's wort was officially approved for use in Germany and went on to become the most popular prescription treatment for mild to moderate depression in that country.

The Symptoms of Mild to Moderate Depression

T o most people, the term *depression* just indicates a dampened mood and pervasive unhappiness. But, actually, depression has many forms and symptoms, and can range from what might best be called a personality style to a catastrophic illness. Some people suffer from significant depression without even knowing it.

This chapter sketches the characteristics of mild to moderate depression (where St. John's wort appears to be useful) and distinguishes it from severe depression (where it is not). These descriptions will help you determine whether St. John's wort might be useful to you or a loved one. However, the apparent extent of depression can be misleading. I strongly recommend seeking a professional evaluation before deciding that your depression is sufficiently mild to warrant herbal, rather than drug, treatment.

Severe Depression Versus Mild to Moderate Depression

Severe major depression is catastrophic. In the words of author William Styron, "It's sadness that has become intensified into excruciating pain." Along with unremitting unhappiness comes paralyzing self-judgment, obsessive guilty rumination, numbness, loss of interest in normal activities, incapacity to deal with life, and recurrent thoughts of death by suicide. The sufferer's life collapses, and suicide becomes an imminent possibility. Severe major depression is often visible in the physical actions of those who suffer from it. Symptoms may include slowed movements, markedly delayed responses to questions, and drawn-out speech. Occasional episodes of frantic activity may arise briefly, only to subside back into leaden slowness.

One might say that in major depression, the emotional structure of the brain freezes into a pattern of misery. It cannot be shaken by any ordinary external event because the computer, so to speak, is locked up. Indeed, one of the earliest successful treatments for major depression was shock therapy, a technique that can be compared to the rebooting of a computer.

Antidepressant drugs are also effective treatments for major depression. Practically any standard pharmaceutical antidepressant has the capacity to lift a person out of depressive collapse, and for this purpose they are indispensable and may even be lifesaving. However, St. John's wort is used for mild to moderate depression, not this terrible emotional illness.

Mild to moderate depression is much less catastrophic. Life may be difficult, but it isn't impossible. Perhaps you feel constantly fatigued, but you succeed in getting out of bed; and though you may feel unhappy, you're not ready to end it all. You probably don't appear particularly depressed to others. Your doctor might still want to give you

Prozac or another drug, but St. John's wort might be equally effective with fewer side effects.

There is no widely accepted definition for mild to moderate depression, and some of the language used can be confusing. In many of the studies that evaluated St. John's wort as a treatment for depression, all participating individuals had been diagnosed with major depression. However, according to a rating scale used by the investigators, the symptoms were not extremely severe (see chapter 5). One might say they suffered from "mild to moderate major depression." Other authorities reserve the term *major depression* for severe symptoms, and use the technical term *dysthymia* for more moderate symptoms. Still others refer to *clinical depression* when they mean *severe major depression.* Since there is no overarching consensus on the right language to use, in this book I will avoid the controversy and simply contrast mild to moderate depression with severe depression.

The apparent extent of depression can be misleading. Seek a professional evaluation before deciding that your depression is sufficiently mild to warrant herbal rather than drug treatment.

Antidepressant drugs were originally invented for severe depression. The problem with using them for mild to moderate depression is that they frequently cause a raft of unpleasant side effects. It's reasonable to put up with a few side effects if you're suicidally depressed. But when depression is only mild to moderate, it isn't quite so sensible to take a drug that can cause anxiety, severe insomnia, or loss of the ability to achieve an orgasm. Because it is essentially side-effect free, St. John's wort may be preferable.

The Symptoms of Mild to Moderate Depression

There are many symptoms of mild to moderate depression. Some of the most common include depressed mood, numbness, irritability, sleep disturbances, and low energy or fatigue.

Depressed Mood

The most obvious symptom of depression is a depressed mood—sadness, gloom, and a sense of pervading melancholy. Feelings of unhappiness float just beneath the surface, ready to attach themselves to any outward event and make you say to yourself, "I told you so! You have every reason to feel miserable." If you experience this kind of depression, you may burst into tears on slight provocation and the future may seem to hold mostly the promise of failure. As one person said to me, "It used to be I could look at my children and feel proud. Now I keep thinking that I'm failing them, and that they'll probably turn out all messed up, like me."

In severe major depression, this mood is overwhelming, unbroken, and often excruciatingly painful; but if your depression is mild to moderate, your unhappiness is not as intense, you have both good and bad days, and most of the time your suffering seems more troublesome than disabling. Thoughts of suicide may flit by, but you have no real inclination to act on them. Also, crying spells almost always occur for a reason, unlike the almost continuous, unexplainable crying that can occur in severe major depression.

A woman whom I shall call Ann suffered from depressed mood. To all outward appearances she was perfectly well-adjusted. She had a happy family and a good job, and only those who knew her well were aware that anything was wrong. But one day Ann confessed her inner feelings to her doctor. "I'm just forcing a smile half the time," she said. "It's like an act I have to keep up. Inside, I often feel like I've just been to a funeral. I don't know why."

Although Ann went to counselors and therapists for years and had thoroughly worked through the few childhood traumas that could be identified, the sadness just wouldn't stop coming. Her doctor suggested antidepressants, but Ann was reluctant at first. "I don't want to be dependent on a drug," she said. It took a while to convince her, but when she finally did take the antidepressant Zoloft she was amazed by the results. "Nothing changed about me except that I didn't feel sad anymore. It was like someone carved away my misery with a knife. I felt bright inside, and didn't have to fake my smile."

Antidepressant drugs were originally invented for severe depression. The problem with using them for mild to moderate depression is that they frequently cause a raft of unpleasant side effects.

Apparently, Ann is one of those people for whom depression stems primarily from a biochemical cause. Psychotherapy had been useful, but it couldn't touch her depressed mood. Drug therapy was a revelation.

Ann soon became a walking advertisement for Zoloft. She told all her friends about how much it had helped her and, for a brief period, she even considered writing a book about it. But within a month she discovered that there was a price to pay for her improvement—in side effects.

She developed diarrhea, headaches, and mild insomnia—all side effects that she could live with. What Ann could not tolerate, however, was the anorgasmia: the complete inability to have an orgasm. She had no trouble becoming aroused, but she "felt like a train all revved up with nowhere to go." Before Zoloft, her sex life had been free from problems. She decided this one side effect was intolerable.

Individuals who are depressed typically possess a low opinion of their own value. A critical voice runs continually in the mind. "You're a nobody." This constant interior disparagement can be very destructive.

She also hated the feeling of being on a drug. "I always feel like there's something foreign in my system, something chemical," she explained. For these two reasons, Ann quit taking Zoloft after a couple of months. Unfortunately, she started to feel sad again almost immediately. "It was like my insides just drained away. The melancholy came right back, like before."

Her psychiatrist suggested the drug Serzone, an antidepressant that typically does not interfere with orgasm. Unfortunately, "Serzone made me a walking zombie." As a third try, Prozac was prescribed but caused horrible insomnia. "I finally decided I'd rather be depressed than put up with all these annoying side effects," she said when she came to me.

It seemed that Ann was a perfect candidate to try St. John's wort. Although she was depressed, she wasn't paralyzed by her depression. Her sadness was uncomfortable, but it wasn't unbearable; and she never felt so badly that she would consider suicide. Thus, Ann fit the picture of mild to moderate depression.

It took about 6 weeks for St. John's wort to achieve full effect. "It came on gently and gradually," Ann said. "The sadness didn't shut off all at once like with Zoloft; it gradually evaporated. I didn't have any side effects, either." What's more, Ann preferred the feeling of taking a natural herb instead of a chemical.

Of course, testimonials such as this one are of no scientific value. One success says nothing about general effectiveness, and, indeed, St. John's wort doesn't always work as well as it did for Ann. The formal research that scientifically evaluates St. John's wort's effectiveness is explored in chapters 5 and 8.

Numbness

Gloom and sadness aren't the only moods associated with depression. For some people, dullness, numbness, and apathy predominate. These symptoms of depression make it difficult to get extremely excited about anything, either good *or* bad. In fact, nothing seems to matter much at all. "I don't really care if I go out on a date or stay home," one patient said. "It's all the same to me."

In mild to moderate depression, this state of numbness isn't absolute. Desires (such as wanting to go out on a date) percolate beneath the surface, but acting on them seems like too much trouble. This is a milder symptom than that which occurs with major depression, where desires seem dead and buried. But the relative apathy of mild to moderate depression is enough to destroy initiative and paralyze activity. As one individual explained, "I can only be bothered to do what I have to do. Occasionally, I do go out for fun, but only when it doesn't require too much effort."

Antidepressants can be quite successful with this form of depression. Caring and interest may come back again, but some people complain that there is an artificial quality to their renewed involvement in life. As one person said, "I go out dancing now, but sometimes it feels like it's the Prozac dancing instead of me." Some people report that

St. John's wort produces a more natural feeling of enthusiasm, although this may simply be due to the positive suggestion produced by the fact that it's an herb rather than a drug.

Irritability

Depressed mood and numbness are immediately recognizable as symptoms of depression. However, there is another symptom that may go unrecognized, even by professionals: irritability. This type of unusual irritability is a common dominant mood in depressed children and adolescents.

Everyone is irritable sometimes (especially teenagers!). Not enough sleep, a rushed schedule, too many responsibilities, or simply "bad days" can cause irritability in the best of us. But the irritability of hidden depression has a quality that psychologists call "overdetermined." It seems to have a life of its own, regardless of whether there are any contributing circumstances that might reasonably be expected to cause it.

The idea that irritability can mask depression is not new, but recent evidence supporting this notion has come through "listening to antidepressants," as Peter Kramer evocatively describes it.

Physicians have observed that when hyperirritable people take antidepressants, they frequently become much calmer. However, antidepressants are not tranquilizers and do not universally produce a sense of calm. The calming effect is remarkably specific to a certain kind of irritability, which has led to thinking that this specific kind of irritability is really depression in disguise.

This reasoning has been criticized as being somewhat circular. Nonetheless, the discovery that hyperirritability often responds to antidepressant treatment has been a great boon to many children and their families. After taking a low dose of antidepressant for a while, behavior, mood, and communication may improve dramatically.

Jason's Story

Jason had always been a rather irritable, grumpy teenager, but 6 months after his parents divorced, it escalated. He was constantly rude to his brothers and sisters, acted like it was a grave personal insult when his mother asked him to take out the garbage, and would curse and swear when it took more than a few seconds for someone to pass him the ketchup at dinner.

His mother at first took this as normal teenage moodiness aggravated by stress. But when she casually mentioned it to her doctor, he proposed giving Jason antidepressants. The only problem was that Jason refused to take them. "I know someone at school on Paxil," he said, "and he's a zombie. No thanks."

He didn't object to St. John's wort, although he was quite sure it wouldn't work. Four weeks later, his mother noticed a dramatic change. "He's back to being the normal surly teenager I'm used to," she said.

While this anecdote illustrates how St. John's wort may be more palatable to teenagers, it can't be taken as evidence of effectiveness. Unfortunately, St. John's wort has not been scientifically studied in children or adolescents.

For children, there is one great advantage to using an herb instead of a drug. Taking a drug seems to send the message "you're sick." Because children respond readily to symbolism, after taking drugs for 1 year or more they may internalize that message and view themselves as basically "broken."

An herbal treatment, however, can be honestly presented as a kind of food. As one psychiatrist said to his 10-year-old patient, "This herb feeds your patience. It makes it stronger." Thinking of yourself as in need of nourishment feels a lot better than believing that you're broken and need to be fixed by taking a drug. It creates a much better self-image. However, the safety of St. John's wort in children has not been established (see chapter 7).

With adolescents, the problem is slightly different. If you tell a teenager that a drug will cure his or her depression, this suggests that drugs are good options for altering mood. For teenagers, the leap from taking a prescription drug to taking an illegal drug may not seem very far. If you give the teenager an herb instead, with its connotations of being a natural, healthful treatment, it is possible to maintain the separation from taking unhealthy illegal drugs.

Sleep Disturbances

Depression can cause either insomnia or the need for excessive sleep. (This is true of both severe depression and the more mild to moderate forms.) When the prevailing symptom is insomnia, it's usually a special kind of insomnia: early morning awakening. You may be able to fall asleep well enough, but somewhere between three and five in the morning you find yourself suddenly wide awake. This puts you in an awkward situation. If you simply get up and get out of bed, you'll feel terrible the rest of the day: exhausted, headachy, and unable to concentrate. If you stay in bed, however, you'll just toss and turn and probably start worrying about something.

Antidepressants can benefit sleep in one of two ways. The older antidepressants, such as amitriptylline and trazodone, cause drowsiness directly and make pretty good sleeping pills. Unfortunately, they can also produce a drugged feeling round-the-clock. Most of them can also cause dramatic weight gain.

The newer antidepressants are not sleeping pills. In fact, many create a stimulating effect that can, at first, make insomnia much worse. Sleeping only begins to prove once the full antidepressant effect sets in, whic may take as long as 4 to 6 weeks. Apparently, the disturbances of brain chemicals that occur in depression also cause early morning awakening. When a better balance is restored through successful drug treatment, sleep improves at the same time.

This effect isn't a sure thing, however. The stimulating side effects of the new antidepressants can be so strong that the net result is to make insomnia far worse. Frequently those individuals for whom insomnia is a part of their depression find that they must take two different antidepressants: one to wake up and another to go to sleep.

For many people, this two-drug approach doesn't feel right. As one patient said to me, "It's like being on uppers and

Every human being is a complex, amazing creature, a walking universe of thoughts, feelings, and talents. But depression can make it very difficult to feel your own richness.

downers. I started to think I was Bob Fosse in *All That Jazz.*"

St. John's wort may at times be a better option for insomnia than conventional antidepressants. It appears to be a "clean" antidepressant that can improve sleep without causing either excessive wakefulness or daytime drowsiness. However, like the newer antidepressants St. John's wort is not a direct sleeping pill. If it is successful, its results will take many weeks to develop. More potent sleep-aids may be necessary for severe insomnia.

prevailing symptom of depression is exces-
ss, different considerations apply. Peter was a
nine who, when depressed, went to bed as
early as en in the evening and would still resent the
alarm clock when it woke him at eight the following morning. He found that Prozac cured his excessive sleeping in
short order, but the effect was too dramatic. He could
only sleep 4 hours a night. Other antidepressants might
have been a better choice. St. John's wort, too, might be
worth considering.

Low Energy or Fatigue

Many individuals visit the doctor's office for the sole complaint of fatigue. Unfortunately, a partial list of the medical diseases that can cause fatigue would fill at least a
page in this book. Attempting a diagnosis can involve a
great number of tests and, in the end, there may still be
no diagnosis.

In many cases, the sensation of fatigue may be due to
problems in the fine-tuning of the body too subtle for
medicine to identify. Sometimes the underlying cause of
tiredness, however, is depression. There is no doubt of the
converse: Depression can certainly cause a pervading
sense of low energy.

Several people who seem to be particularly perceptive
about their own sensations have told me that the fatigue
of depression has a unique character. "It seems to have its
roots in my soul," one said. "I'm weary like I've just been
through a battle." Another person explained it this way:
"Children have a connection to heaven that makes them
bounce, and, although it gradually fades, a healthy grown-
up shouldn't have lost it all. But I have no bounce. I have
to use my will when love should be enough."

There may be a brief burst of energy in the morning or
evening, but patients with depression-induced fatigue drag
through most of the day. Even play may come to feel like

work. People suffering from severe depression often can't even get out of bed, but in mild to moderate depression tiredness is a problem, not a master. You may wake up tired and find that exercise fails to give you a boost; and, whether it's work or play, all your activities are hampered by a chronic feeling that you just don't have enough energy.

Depression-induced fatigue typically responds very well to the Prozac class of drugs. One of the most common statements I hear from individuals who take these medications is that they feel energized. As one patient said, "I used to be running on fumes, but now I feel like I have gas in the tank." Both work and play may become easier and more enjoyable when you have enough *oomph* to carry them through with enthusiasm. St. John's wort may be an excellent option too.

Low Self-Esteem

Patients who are depressed typically possess a low opinion of their own value. A critical voice runs continually in the mind, providing an unwanted commentary on everything they do. "There you go, blowing it as usual. Why bother trying to do that; you'll fail. Don't talk to *them;* why would they be interested in *you?* You're a nobody." This constant internal disparagement can be very destructive.

One of the worst characteristics of low self-esteem is that it's self-reinforcing. For example, if I believe that I can't possibly get a good job, I won't even bother applying; or if I do apply, I'll convey by word and body language that no sensible employer would ever want to hire me. Unless an employer takes me on out of a sense of charity, I'll probably end up with jobs that I am overqualified for or that no one else wants to take. The inner critic will then take my misfortune for an opportunity. "See? You're no good," it will say. "Look at the kind of work you have to do. It just goes to show how worthless you are."

This is really very unfair, because it was the inner critic itself that caused the problem in the first place. But inner critics are seldom fair. Although they frequently pretend to have our best interests at heart ("I'm only telling you this for your own good"), it's all a sham. Sometimes, the inner critic seems to have no greater aim than to cause unhappiness.

Low self-esteem interferes with relationships just as much as with jobs. As one person said to me, "I don't bother trying to go out with men I really like, because they seem out of reach. The way I feel, you'd think this was the 1800s and I was a peasant in love with an aristocrat. The good ones seem 'above me' or 'out of my league.' It isn't logical, but that's how it goes. So I pursue guys who I really don't like. I don't seem to think I'm good enough unless the guy's a low-life."

In many cases low self-esteem is brought on by problems in childhood. The inner critic is often a carbon copy of parents or siblings who used constant shaming as a tool. A good psychotherapist can help us understand the origin of the inner critic, separate ourselves from its voice, and provide an alternative stream of positive mental commentary. But this approach isn't always completely successful. Sometimes, it seems that brain chemicals become so poisoned that no amount of positive self-encouragement can make a difference.

It is in this condition that antidepressant therapy can be particularly helpful. Drugs seem to push the inner critic into the background, where it can be managed more easily. As one person said to me, "The critical voice is still there, but it's not right in my face. It's somewhere across the room now. I don't have to listen to it." St. John's wort may be able to provide the same benefit.

Poor Concentration or
Difficulty Making Decisions

Depression can make simple tasks and decision making much more difficult. It's like there's an undertow. The constant drag of depression interferes with your thinking processes. You mix up simple instructions, go Thursday to a Friday appointment, or go to the store and not remember why. You can't decide whether to buy the wool sweater or the cotton sweater, because your inner critic gets in the way and informs you that whatever you decide will be wrong. In severe major depression, even the simplest decision may seem impossible.

Successful treatment of depression alleviates this symptom. When depression is no longer grumbling away in the depths, your mind breaks free from its troubling preoccupations and can get down to business. One person said to me, "When I got over being depressed, it seemed like my IQ jumped 20 points."

Unfortunately, antidepressant drugs can cause mental confusion, memory loss, and a sense of disorientation as direct side effects. Common descriptions include: "I feel scatterbrained," "I can't remember anything," and "Half the time I don't even know where I am." In such cases, St. John's wort may be a better choice. It doesn't seem to have any adverse mental effects, so its benefits for depression are not counteracted by drug-induced confusion.

Feelings of Hopelessness

Hope is one of the most universal of human needs, but in depression it's severely lacking. Under normal circumstances, each morning brings some optimism. No matter how dark the future seemed last night, when the sun comes up, more options seem possible than you previously thought. But depression can take away much of this natural rejuvenation. The morning may bring with it no more enthusiasm than the night before, and you may have to get by on mere dogged persistence.

While individuals with major depression frequently lose all hope and turn to suicide, in mild to moderate depression, there is enough hope to get by. However, there is not as much as there should be. One of the first signs of improving depression is a renewed sense of possibilities in life. Any successful treatment for depression can produce this positive result, whether psychotherapy, antidepressant drugs, or St. John's wort.

Eating Disorders

The effect of depression on eating habits can go either one of two ways. Some people overeat to compensate for their unhappiness, while others lose interest in food.

The most common of these possibilities is the familiar eating-for-comfort that can also occur without accompanying depression. When depression is involved, recovery from the depression will tend to normalize eating habits. However, most of the antidepressants in common use prior to Prozac often directly cause weight gain and an increase in appetite. Amitriptylline is one of the worst; weight increases of over 20 pounds are not uncommon during treatment with this somewhat outdated medication.

Drugs in the Prozac family are much better in this regard. Not only do they not cause weight gain as a side effect, but in many cases they directly promote weight loss. This effect, is discussed in *Safer Than Phen-Fen!* by Michael Anchors (Prima, 1997). It doesn't appear likely that the use of St. John's wort will provide any similar benefit with regard to weight loss, other than through its effect on depression.

But when the eating disturbance caused by depression is loss of interest in food, Prozac-type drugs can be an obstacle. St. John's wort, with its lack of side effects, may help to restore appetite more effectively.

Emptiness

Depression brings with it a kind of inner emptiness or hollowness. All people experience a sense of emptiness from time to time, but depression amplifies this normal human experience. As one individual said, "I feel that if someone could see inside me, they'd find that there's not much there."

Of course, this sensation is an illusion. Every human being is a complex, amazing creature, a walking universe of thoughts, feelings, and talents. But depression can make it very difficult to feel your own richness. If depressed, even when others find you charming and interesting, you may wonder what they see in you (if you let yourself recognize their appreciation at all).

One of the first signs of recovery from depression is a feeling of being more filled-up inside. Any of the numerous treatments for depression can help produce this result, including St. John's wort. However, the herb will not be effective in severe major depression, where the emptiness can be so great that, as one person said, "I feel like the hole inside me could swallow the world." When it's that bad, drug treatment is necessary.

Anxiety

Anxiety can be a disease all in its own right, but it frequently accompanies depression. Of course, life is anxiety-provoking in general. When anxiety becomes excessive, or when it detaches itself from real concerns and floats through your mental life like an ever-present cloud, that's when it is a real problem. One person described the feeling like this: "I'm always sure disaster is just around the corner." Depression magnifies anxiety by decreasing your natural defenses against it.

The anxiety of mild to moderate depression can be pervasive, annoying, and continuous. You feel that you are always on edge, always expecting something bad to happen. You don't seem to be able to relax like other people, and you wish your nerves would simply take a vacation. However, these symptoms are less intense than the severe, almost disabling anxiety that may accompany major depression.

In some cases anxiety gives rise to panic attacks. These can produce such severe heart pounding, chest pressure, and sense of impending doom that they may be confused with symptoms of a heart attack.

Antidepressants have proved to be useful treatments for anxiety. However, it is their long-term antidepressant effect that relieves symptoms. In the short term, most of the newer antidepressants have a disturbing potential to increase anxiety. Individuals who are already anxious seldom appreciate being told that a medication may make them feel worse for a month or so.

St. John's wort, with its virtual absence of side effects, can be a useful alternate choice. However, the herb is not sufficient treatment for severe anxiety, nor does it work for panic attacks. Recently, a physician called me up wanting me to talk her patient out of taking St. John's wort. "She's highly agitated," the physician said. "She scans the room when she's in my office, wakes up at night with panic attacks, and her husband says she paces back and forth at dinner."

I agreed that St. John's wort was not the right approach for this woman. At best it would be too mild and too subtle. She probably needed quick-acting drug medication. This is because intense anxiety requires more aggressive treatment than St. John's wort can provide. Even for relatively mild chronic anxiety, many alternative physicians combine a natural antianxiety treatment with St. John's wort to enhance and speed effectiveness, such as described in chapter 9. However, the safety of such combinations has not been proven.

Guilt

Actor and director Woody Allen has made an art of guilt, but the symptoms he presents in exaggerated forms are immediately recognizable to anyone who suffers from depression. That nagging sense that you've done something wrong, obsession with past errors, and overscrupulous concern about hurting someone's feelings: All of these go along with depression almost as inevitably as depressed mood.

Like so many symptoms of depression, guilt in itself is not an illness. If we never felt guilt (or the related emotion, shame), we would all behave as selfishly as 2 year olds. But in depression, guilt is overdetermined. The guilt is free-floating, waiting for an event to which it can attach. Guilt feelings usually, but not always, retreat to manageable levels as depression is resolved. St. John's wort may be as helpful here as standard antidepressants so long as the underlying depression isn't too severe.

Obsession with Body Symptoms

Many people who are depressed find that they spend altogether too much time focusing on body symptoms. A mild spell of constipation, a headache, or a stiff neck can take on significance all out of proportion to the actual discomfort. There are many factors behind this commonly observed phenomenon. Because depression limits interest in our external lives, internal phenomena begin to loom larger. When depressed, we also have fewer inner resources to cope with discomfort and therefore succumb more easily. In addition, the anxiety associated with depression can give rise to terrible fantasies of cancer and imminent death, causing our minds to dwell on symptoms and our imaginations to amplify them.

Furthermore, there seems to be a direct relationship between depression and pain, as if the brain chemicals involved in each are similar. Many people with chronic pain experience a marked improvement after starting antidepressant therapy. Unfortunately, medical doctors sometimes turn this observation around and make a weapon of it. For example, if a person doesn't recover from a whiplash injury in the time the doctor expects, the physician may use what he knows about depression to shift

Mike's Story

Mike was a 45-year-old man with a very high-stress job. It was his responsibility to make sure that highway repair projects in a major city didn't cause major disruptions of traffic flow. What this really amounted to was fending off the anger of innumerable businesses and commuters. Every time I saw him, I ended up grateful that I didn't have to deal with such no-win propositions myself.

He came to me for severe chronic shoulder pain. In succession, I had him try every treatment I knew—acupuncture, chiropractic care, osteopathy, massage, and pain medications. Strangely, nothing worked. Everyone he saw reported back that they couldn't find much wrong with him.

Finally, I suggested that he try an antidepressant. He angrily told me that he wasn't depressed and didn't need one. I agreed that he didn't seem depressed, but pointed out that I couldn't think of anything else to try. "I know it sounds far-

blame. Too many individuals are told, "You don't have any pain; you're just depressed."

This is an unfortunate distortion of the real situation. Just because depression amplifies discomfort doesn't mean the pain is "all in your head," and I sincerely wish doctors would quit using that expression. It is demeaning, hurtful, and ultimately useless.

Nonetheless, antidepressant medication can be quite helpful in dealing with pain. Whether the effect is due to changing brain chemicals, or simply to the fact that with an elevated mood it's easier to deal with pain, such treatment fetched," I said, "but maybe you actually just have a little bit of discomfort and your depression is amplifying it." This made him even angrier, and I couldn't blame him. It sounded to him like I was saying, "It's all in your head." His own experience told him it was all in his shoulder, not his head.

But after he calmed down, Mike decided to try it. "Who knows," he shrugged, "maybe it will help my stress level anyway."

We were both surprised by how well it worked. After 6 weeks on Prozac, his shoulder stopped bothering him. "It's still a little sore," he said, "but I mean just a little. It's nothing really. I don't know why it used to drive me so crazy."

This story shouldn't be used to suggest that most pain is due to depression. The overwhelming majority of painful shoulders, for example, are caused by muscle injuries. But depression can sometimes be the major cause of any kind of pain. St. John's wort may be a useful option.

can often help. A small study reported in 1994 showed that St. John's wort can help relieve the physical discomfort associated with depression too.[1] In this trial, 39 participants whose depression included many physical complaints were treated with either St. John's wort or placebo. Even those taking placebo improved (as always), but those given the herb improved significantly more.

Difficulty Managing Stress

Few of us handle stress particularly well, but depression turns "difficult" into "almost impossible." What other people find merely unpleasant, you may find almost impossible to manage. The multiple demands, interruptions, and irritations of work and family life may seem overwhelming. If you were in a severe major depression, they really would overwhelm you, and you'd probably fail to manage them altogether. But in mild to moderate depression you cope, yet only by working a lot harder than you feel you should need to.

On reflection, this shouldn't be surprising. When you suffer from depression, part of your brain is always busy processing guilt feelings, scanning for rejection, and expecting the worst. Have you ever used a computer that's trying to perform two tasks at the same time, such as print a document while running another program? The main program may slow to a crawl because the computer has to use part of its "brain" to concentrate on printing. Something similar happens when you are depressed. You lack the resources to deal with life's stresses successfully because much of your brain is occupied elsewhere.

In such a situation, successful treatment of depression by any route may make managing stress easier. Many people say that antidepressants give them increased reserve capacity and a greater ability to stay calm in the midst of many demands. Unfortunately, the usefulness of conventional antidepressants is somewhat diminished by the side effects of drowsiness or agitation. Side-effect–free St. John's wort may once more be a better choice.

Hidden Forms of Depression

Besides the direct symptoms of depression presented, there are several personality traits that psychologists have begun to suspect might represent depression in disguise. This impression has developed as a consequence of "listening to antidepressants," as mentioned in the description of irritability. In perhaps 1 of 20 cases, people who take Prozac and other drugs experience what amounts to a remake of personality. Such traits as shyness, excessive caution, timidity, and fear of rejection sometimes dramatically change. Some physicians have concluded that some features of personality might actually be identical to depression in a biochemical sense.

It is also possible, however, that an underlying depression is simply exacerbating a personality trait that exists for other reasons. When the depression diminishes, other parts of the personality can come to the fore. Other authorities point out that cocaine and alcohol can also reduce shyness. Maybe Prozac changes personality as a lucky side effect.

The effects of Prozac on personality is a discussion in progress. But one fact isn't controversial: Depression can certainly contribute to personal difficulties of any kind, especially the following ones listed.

Excessive Shyness

A depressed person has to battle inner voices making such unpleasant comments as "You're unattractive," "You sound stupid," and "No one would want to listen to you." Who wouldn't be shy under those circumstances? One response to such inner voices is to avoid situations that trigger them.

I remember one young woman in her 20s who was so shy she didn't dare take a job that required contact with the public. What Lisa really wanted to do was become a veterinarian, because she loved animals, but she knew she couldn't face the interview process necessary to get into school. She took a low-paying job as an assistant bookkeeper instead, because it allowed her to hide.

Years of psychotherapy had helped Lisa understand why she felt this way, but it was only when she took Prozac that she could overcome her fears. She still had to work at it, but drug treatment was a useful and important step forward for her.

Unfortunately, along with its boost, Prozac gave her diarrhea, heart palpitations, and headaches. Other antidepressants caused similarly intolerable side effects. When she finally tried St. John's wort, Lisa found a treatment she could live with. With the help of St. John's wort and the skills she had learned in psychotherapy, she found herself equal to the task of overcoming her fears.

How much of it was St. John's wort and how much was the psychotherapy? Honestly, I don't know. Until there is good research, we will not really know whether St. John's wort (or Prozac) has any effect on personality traits such as shyness.

Oversensitivity to Rejection

Extreme sensitivity to rejection and other emotionally unpleasant experiences may also represent a covert form of depression in some people. Of course, none of us like to be rejected, but in order to have a social life, we find it necessary to take that risk. Only by staying home alone all the time can we completely eliminate the possibility that someone may express dislike for our company.

For some people, however, never leaving home sounds pretty good. You may be so sensitive to rejection that you would rather face loneliness and social isolation than run any risk of experiencing what could be a catastrophically painful event.

I remember a 35-year-old man who had remained single all of his life. At the first hint of displeasure from a potential partner, he wanted to run. As he described it, "I just don't have enough of myself inside me to handle rejection. If I get a hint that a woman is going to show she doesn't like me, I start to feel like I don't exist. When I actually do get rejected, it hurts worse than a broken bone. I feel like I'm dying."

Rejection isn't the only form of unpleasant emotional experience that can cause depressed people to "crash."

Mild criticism from a bank teller, a bad grade in school, or even a rude honk in traffic can be enough to provoke a painful and prolonged response in those who are excessively thin-skinned. Very likely, depression plays a role for many people who suffer from these extreme emotional reactions, and any proven treatment for depression will provide at least some relief.

Lack of Assertiveness

Depression can also get in the way of assertiveness. As one woman said to me, "How can I stand up for myself when I think I'm nobody?" She would act like a doormat most of the time and then suddenly explode with resentment.

Psychologists speak of finding the midway point between aggression and passivity. As depression improves, this point of healthy assertiveness may become much easier to achieve. Psychotherapy is probably the most helpful treatment here, but occasionally Prozac seems to spectacularly increase assertiveness all by itself. I have not heard any reports of similarly dramatic results produced by St. John's wort.

Inability to Take Risks

Life involves numerous risks. Unless we are willing to run the risk of failing we can't succeed: a cliché that is nonetheless true. But some people find it very difficult to take any risks at all. They feel compelled to choose the most cautious course at every decision point in life. Of course, cautiousness is not a disease. The continuum that goes from excessive caution to excessive risk-taking includes a wide spectrum that is normal.

But some people are so cautious that it is more of a problem than a simple personality trait. They may feel a strong desire to take more risks but feel an inner compulsion against it. This excessive cautiousness may very well be a symptom of depression.

It isn't difficult to understand how a general sense of gloominess and negativity would raise the stakes in any form of risky behavior. Overcautiousness may thus respond well to antidepressant treatment. Psychotherapy is usually essential as well.

There are many more possible manifestations and variations to the symptoms of depression. But this brief introduction allows us to turn to theories of what causes depression.

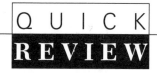

QUICK REVIEW

- Depression has many forms and symptoms. In its most severe form, depression can lead to physical slowing down, an inability to cope with life, and the very real risk of suicide.

- St. John's wort is not appropriate for severe depression. Seek professional consultation to make sure you do not suffer from severe depression before using this herbal treatment.

- Symptoms of mild to moderate depression include depressed mood, numbness, irritability, sleep disturbances (either too much or too little), loss of energy, low self-esteem, poor concentration, difficulty making decisions, feelings of hopelessness, disruption of eating (excessive eating or loss of appetite), anxiety, a sensation of emptiness inside, guilt, obsession with body symptoms, and difficulty managing stress.

- Like standard antidepressants, St. John's wort may be helpful for many aspects of mild to moderate depression.

What Causes Depression?

Depression does not have one single cause. Actually, no complex problem has one single cause or cure, whether it's the high divorce rate in the United States or the conflicts in the Middle East. Attempts throughout history to understand depression have led to a variety of theories and suggested treatments. These approaches can be understood, however, as a swing back and forth between two basic stances: viewing depression as a problem either in the "software" or in the "hardware" of the brain.

Computers require both software and hardware to run effectively. Software theories of depression look to the thoughts and feelings produced by actions, intentions, and experiences, whereas hardware theories focus on the physical structures of the brain and body themselves. In reality, both approaches have validity and enduring significance.

Ancient Theories of Depression

Perhaps the earliest "software" explanation for depression invoked the influence of deities or spirits. In her wonderful biography of Alexander the Great, *Fire from Heaven,* author Mary Renault shows how ancient Greeks attributed their moods to the active intervention of their gods. When Alexander felt confidence and power, he assumed that Hercules was infusing his soul with divine energy; but when he fell into despondency, he presumed that his actions had offended one or another of the deities he believed ruled his life.

Like all theories, this explanation for depression led to certain lines of "treatment." An ancient Greek afflicted with prolonged despondency might very well have felt impelled to make a sacrifice to the gods, consult with the Oracle at Delphi, or make a change in plans or behavior. Thus religious action may be considered one of the earliest treatments for depression, and there is no doubt that it frequently succeeds, even today. Modern worshippers may experience a profound uplifting of the spirit after engaging in prayer or other religious rituals. But this was not the only Greek attitude toward depression.

The Four Humors

The ancient Greeks had another perspective on depression as well, one that falls into the "hardware" category. This perspective came out of the dominant scientific approach to medicine of the day, the theory of humors. Although it sounds preposterous now, the humor theory of medicine was the foundation of Hippocrates' approach to healing, and it continued to influence the practice of medicine up through the nineteenth century.

According to this theory, four "humors" constantly flow through the body. Hippocrates called them yellow bile, blood, phlegm, and black bile. A state of balance among these subtle substances is supposed to produce health, while a loss of balance initiates disease. In a state of perfect balance of the humors, perfect equanimity and health would result.

An excess of a particular humor was believed to produce not only physical illness, but also certain characteristic emotional tendencies or temperaments. Respectively, these were described as choleric (angry), sanguine (emotional), phlegmatic (slow to respond), and melancholic (sad). Each of these names has its origin in the associated humor. For example, *melancholy* literally means black bile, because the Greek words for black and bile are *melan* and *cholia.*

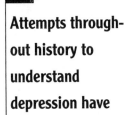

Attempts throughout history to understand depression have led to a variety of theories and suggested treatments.

Thus, in the humor system of illness, depression is a result of too much black bile. Appropriate treatment for depression under this system would aim not so much at curing the symptoms of depression, but at reducing the level of black bile to normal, perhaps raising the other humors at the same time.

The humoral approach to health was still a dominant influence on conventional medicine in nineteenth-century Europe and America. Doctors of that day used leeching to "remove heat from the blood." And when a physician of the nineteenth century recommended a commonsense treatment for depression, such as spending more time outdoors, taking a vacation, or moving to a different climate, he would couch this advice in terms of its good effect on the humors.

But competing theories of depression that fit more into the software category also flourished. One of them, the psychological approach, eventually came to dominate.

Back to Software

In medieval Europe, depression was often attributed to the influence of demonic forces. These supernatural powers were believed capable of entering a human being and producing unexplainable moods and evil actions. One remedy for this was prayer and fasting, another was exorcism, and in the popular mind at least, St. John's wort was also believed to have the power to block such dark influences. As described in chapter 1, this attitude may have reflected an appreciation of the herb's antidepressant effects.

Although the demonic theory of depression passed away long ago, its influence lingers in at least one respect: prejudice toward those who are unlucky enough to suffer from severe depression. Another hangover of the old association between emotional illness and evil was the punitive nature of medical treatments for depression—such as indiscriminate shock treatment—that persisted until a scant three decades ago.

Another software approach to depression grew out of classical Christian theology. This is the idea that sin can eat away at a person's soul if it remains locked up and kept secret. The traditional cure for this interior illness was confession, a potentially marvelous religious practice, the healing power of which is indisputable.

From the confession box, it was only a small step to the client-therapist relationship. Psychotherapy can be seen as a form of confession, in which emotional conflicts unknown even to the patient are brought into the light. But where Christianity focused primarily on sin, psychotherapy devotes its main attention to childhood traumas.

The insights of psychology have taught us the terrible lingering effects of sexual, physical, and emotional abuse suffered during childhood. Treatment for these problems includes individual psychotherapy, group therapy, and self-help practices such as "nurturing the inner child."

However, childhood traumas are not the only psychological cause of depression. Social psychology has demonstrated that poverty, lack of social support, and external stressors such as divorce can cause depression. Cognitive psychology has investigated the relationship between depression's negative self-talk ("I'm no good") and invented treatments that emphasize deliberate positive internal dialogue. For example, a client might be encouraged to say, "I'm a good person who deserves love and success."

These and other psychological viewpoints have been tremendously influential and, until recently, were the dominant paradigm for analyzing depression. But in recent years the pendulum has swung again. The physical side of depression is once more center stage.

The Rise of the Amine Hypothesis

The new hardware approach to depression is officially called the *amine hypothesis.* Since its proposal a few decades ago, it has revolutionized attitudes toward depression.

The amine hypothesis states that depression is caused by low levels of certain brain chemicals, called *amines* (because of their chemical similarity to ammonia). Some of the most famous of these amines are serotonin, norepinephrine, and dopamine. According to the amine hypothesis, depression is the result of low levels of these amines.

It was Prozac that brought this theory into public awareness, but the story really goes back to the 1950s and the drug iproniazid. Iproniazid was initially developed for tuberculosis. However, in 1957 scientists discovered that the drug incidentally helped individuals overcome major depression as well. The effects were sometimes remarkable. People who had been so depressed that they were essentially nonfunctional for years woke up out of their torpor and returned to life. There are some who still doubt that antidepressants actually work, but once you have seen the results in those who were severely depressed you will no longer doubt the effectiveness of these medications. In fact, iproniazid was such an effective antidepressant that within a year it was prescribed to 400,000 individuals. It was the first drug of a class later known as the MAO inhibitors.

Perhaps the earliest explanation for depression invoked the influence of deities or spirits.

At the time of this accidental discovery, scientists were already aware that certain amines had the power to influence blood pressure, heart rate, and wakefulness. They knew that the body manufactures these chemicals for its own purposes and then destroys them or reabsorbs them when they've done their job.

When the antidepressant effects of iproniazid were discovered, scientists began to examine its chemical effects in the brain. This investigation soon revealed that iproniazid raises the levels of these biologically active amines, although in an indirect way. It inhibits the enzyme monoamine-oxidase (hence the name monoamine-oxidase inhibitor, or MAO inhibitor for short). The job of monoamine-oxidase is to break down spare amines. When monoamine-oxidase is inhibited by iproniazid, these amines start to build up in higher concentrations.

This bit of information seemed to suggest that depression might actually be caused by a shortage of amines. The idea made sense because some of these amines were known to be used by the nervous system to transmit its signals. Scientists reasoned that a slowdown of the nervous system caused by low amine levels might tend to depress the brain's functions and cause the symptoms of depression. By artificially raising the levels of neurotransmitters, iproniazid would thereby overcome these symptoms.

This altogether sensible idea was given further impetus with the discovery of a new antidepressant, imipramine. Imipramine doesn't inhibit MAO. Scientists investigating its effects were delighted to discover, however, that imipramine has its own way of raising amine levels. Ordi-

The ancient Greeks had another perspective on depression: the theory of humors.

narily, nerve endings send amines across the small distance of a synapse (a communicating junction between neurons) and then reabsorb those amines once the message has been received. This is another method the body uses to prevent amines from building up to excessive levels. But imipramine blocks this reabsorption, the net result being a rise in the levels of norepinephrine and serotonin, and an improvement in depression. The pattern seemed compelling.

A further observation clinched the hypothesis. The blood-pressure–lowering drug reserpine was already known to make some people become depressed. Medical investigators were very excited when they discovered that reserpine decreases the level of amines in the brain. Again, low amine levels equals depression. The amine hypothesis was on a roll.

St. John's wort, too, was scientifically investigated for its influence on brain chemicals. (The results of this research are discussed in chapter 5.) Pharmaceutical companies synthesized new antidepressants that functioned as designer drugs aimed at specific neurotransmitters. More and more people began to take antidepressant medications with good results, and very soon, hardware theories of depression were back on top. Not since the humor theory of medicine had depression been considered a disease of the body itself.

One significant benefit of this revived focus on the physical was to diminish the stigma of depression. Since the Middle Ages, depressed people had had to contend with the additional insult of being considered lazy, crazy, or possessed. With the advent of the amine hypothesis, however, depression could be conceptualized as a "real" illness, a chemical deficiency like diabetes or hypothyroidism.

Depression clearly is a real illness, and brain chemicals are indisputably involved. Nonetheless, the amine hypothesis has some serious problems too.

Flaws in the Amine Hypothesis

Despite the impressive evidence behind it and the drugs it has inspired, the amine hypothesis is clearly not quite right. For one thing, antidepressant drugs raise the levels of biological amines in a few days, at most, and yet the antidepressant effects of these drugs take weeks to emerge. What is going on during this time lag?

Another problem is that different antidepressants, while affecting different amines, seem to relieve depression just as well as each other. Some drugs raise serotonin levels; others impact norepinephrine. These are very different chemicals, and it's difficult to accept that they could be interchangeable. To make matters even more confusing, the drug buproprion (Wellbutrin) does not significantly affect norepinephrine or serotonin levels but still works as well as Prozac—some might even say better.

Finally, there is no evidence that the brains of depressed people are low in serotonin. Obviously, part of the picture is missing here. Upon reflection, this shouldn't be

We're Still Learning

It's a human tendency to believe that everything has a good explanation. We especially wish to believe that doctors know precisely what they are doing. This is probably the reason why most news reports imply that we understand exactly how Prozac and similar drugs relieve depression. But we don't. In medicine, at least, it is fair to say that our ignorance far exceeds our knowledge.

Antidepressants aren't the only drugs we don't fully understand. For example, if you look up common anti-inflammatory drugs such as Aleve in the Physicians' Drug Reference (PDR), you'll find a disclaimer admitting that their mechanism of action remains unknown.

---

too surprising. There are thousands of active chemicals in the brain. Maybe antidepressants produce their effect by indirectly influencing the levels of as-yet-unidentified chemicals—altering the soup, so to speak, in ways we don't yet understand. Some researchers suspect a role for endorphins and many other specific hormones. However, this all remains speculation.

Unrecognized chemicals aren't the only complication. Scientists have recently discovered that the brain possesses many different kinds of receptors for serotonin and norepinephrine. Antidepressants seem to alter some of these receptors more than others, thereby producing different effects in different parts of the brain. It may be the changed *distribution* of brain chemicals and not their *quantity* that matters most in depression. But this, too, is only a theory.

It will undoubtedly be a long, long time before brain chemistry is fully understood. In the meantime, the truth is that we really don't know how antidepressants (either drug or herbal) work.

And we shouldn't turn our back on software theories, either.

The Big Picture

Realistically, depression is the result of a combination of influences. Traumatic childhood, biological amines, repressed memories, unrecognized brain chemicals, negative self-talk, and special amine receptor sites; all are probably important and mutually influencing. Prozac can facilitate psychotherapy, and psychotherapy can probably raise serotonin levels. The body is all of a piece.

To illustrate the interdependence of causes in depression, I like to use the following analogy. Imagine a car driving on a road littered with nails. The car will probably move rather slowly as the driver tries to steer around the nails. If there are enough nails, however, one will finally puncture a tire, and the car will come to a stop.

In this analogy, it is clearly the nails on the road that are causing the problem. Nonetheless, two cars going down the same road will experience different results. It depends to a great extent on the ruggedness of their tires. Weak tires may suffer a puncture even if there are only a few dull, short nails on the road. But strong tires built with thick layers of rubber and steel can survive all but the biggest, nastiest spikes.

Thus both internal and external factors matter. And if a car should break down in the middle of such a road, two different kinds of "treatments" would apply. The tires would have to be repaired, but the nails should be removed from the road, as well. Taking care of only one side of this equation will produce temporary relief, at best. The cause of the problem is in the car and on the road; both must be treated for good results.

This story is an allegory of depression. If you grew up in a dysfunctional household, you spent most of your early life "driving carefully" to avoid the spikes of abuse. In order to survive, you had to expend a lot of extra energy, and it inhibited you from living a fully normal life.

Eventually, however, you were injured to some extent. Abusive and shaming words, perhaps even physical and sexual abuse came your way, and you suffered from it. But how much you suffered depended to a great extent on how you were constituted physically. Like the cars in the story, some people are more susceptible to emotional injury than others.

Psychological viewpoints have been tremendously influential and, until recently, were the dominant paradigm for analyzing depression.

We have all met people who grew up in horrible environments but turned out pretty well, and others who came from decent homes but developed serious emotional problems anyway. This is because of the "tire" side of the equation. People are gifted with widely varying genetic backgrounds. Some sets of genes provide tremendous resiliency. Others make a person susceptible to developing depression under the slightest provocation.

Of course, the body is far more complex and sophisticated than an automobile. Unlike a machine, the body has the potential to heal itself. With successful psychotherapy, or even sheer personal determination, the brain may adjust its own brain chemicals and eliminate the symptoms of depression. However, it isn't easy, and if genetic influences toward depression are too strong, it simply can't be done.

It is here that antidepressants can be useful. By improving the balance of brain chemicals, antidepressants work on the "tire" side of the equation. With increased energy and elevated mood, everything will become easier. You may gain greater success in psychotherapy and an enhanced ability to make positive life changes. Maybe you will be able to start exercising more, getting out more, eating better, taking on hobbies you enjoy, and developing better relationships. Once on an upward path, there is a win-win cycle. Like standard antidepressants, St. John's wort may be able to help initiate it.

The amine hypothesis states that depression is caused by low levels of certain brain chemicals— called *amines*— such as, serotonin, norepinephrine, and dopamine.

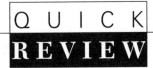

QUICK
REVIEW

- There are many causes of depression. The events of your life from early childhood on undoubtedly play a major role. But other factors in depression may be more physical in nature.

- Recently, the role of brain chemistry in depression has taken center stage due to the dramatic effects of antidepressant drugs in severe major depression.

- According to the amine hypothesis, depression is due to an imbalance in the levels of a family of chemicals called biological amines.

- Serotonin is the most famous of the biological amines. Prozac raises serotonin levels, and it is widely assumed that this is the explanation for its antidepressant effects. However, there are many problems with this hypothesis.

- Contrary to popular belief, we don't really understand how Prozac or any other antidepressant actually works.

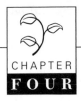

Conventional Treatment for Depression

Antidepressant drugs have provided enormous benefits to millions of depressed people. In this chapter we look at some of the benefits and risks of these important medications.

As mentioned earlier, the story of antidepressant drugs begins with iproniazid, an antituberculosis drug found quite by accident to improve depression. Iproniazid was taken off the market after reports that it could cause jaundice circulated. (Ironically, the reports were probably erroneous.) However, in its short tenure iproniazid had been so remarkably effective that a search for replacements began in earnest. This effort soon led to two large classes of antidepressants that were to dominate the field for decades: the MAO inhibitors, which work like iproniazid, and the tricyclics, of which imipramine was the first representative.

These early drugs were effective antidepressants but they proved to cause numerous side effects and toxicities. In an attempt to minimize such problems, researchers looked for ways to make the drugs' actions more specific.

MAO inhibitors and, to a lesser extent, drugs are medical shotguns, raising the le amines at the same time. Scientists reasoned only one of the amines mattered with respect to depression and that changing levels of other amines only caused side effects. By seeking to develop drugs that would work on only one chemical at a time, they hoped that they might be able to create a clean medication that would relieve depression and do nothing else.

This was the origin of the selective serotonin-reuptake inhibitors, or SSRIs. This class of drugs, of which Prozac is the most famous representative, specifically raises serotonin levels without affecting other major amines. During their development, the SSRIs proved to be potent antidepressants and far less dangerous when taken in overdose than their predecessors. However, the Holy Grail of zero side effects has not yet been achieved. The search for side-effect–free antidepressants continues.

Prozac: The Most Popular Antidepressant in History

Prozac was the first of the SSRIs to be developed, closely followed by Zoloft and Paxil. It was the drug that made antidepressants wildly popular, and it remains the most widely prescribed antidepressant drug in history. Prozac's appeal lies in its energizing characteristics.

The tricyclic class of antidepressants is plagued by two major side effects that sharply decrease its usefulness in treating depression: fatigue and sleepiness. Because a sense of low energy is one of the defining characteristics of depression, a drug that lowers energy has a major strike against it. In catastrophic major depression it is possible to overlook this side effect, because the disease symptoms are overwhelming. But for mild to moderate depression, a medication that causes severe fatigue is next to useless.

Most tricyclic drugs produce so much drowsiness that they make excellent sleeping pills. It can be difficult to carry out the activities of daily life while taking them, and indeed their labeling warns against driving or operating heavy machinery. The prospect of sleeping through life may appeal to some, but most people suffering from depression would rather engage life more fully and successfully. Hence the great contribution of Prozac. While matching the antidepressant powers of the tricyclic drugs, it simultaneously produces for many people an enhanced sense of energy and alertness—a combination that made Prozac a stunning overnight success.

The Holy Grail of zero side effects has not yet been achieved. The search for side-effect–free antidepressants continues.

Prozac was the first widely available drug truly useful for mild to moderate depression. Millions of people who previously chose to remain untreated because they could not accept the side effects of existing medications found in Prozac a wonderful opportunity for improving their lives.

No drug is perfect, however. After a while, reports began to come back revealing that the strength of Prozac was also a weakness. Along with increased energy came frequent reports of insomnia, restlessness, agitation, irritability, anxiety, dry mouth, sweating, and palpitations: symptoms, in other words, of excess stimulation.

In those for whom insomnia is a part of depression, the drawbacks of Prozac may be evident from the first dose. Falling asleep typically becomes more difficult, and the familiar symptom of early morning awakening grows increasingly intense. As with use of any stimulant, missed sleep may not seem to matter at first. People who have just started taking Prozac say they feel alert and energetic even though they aren't sleeping well. However, after a while the lack of sleep begins to take its toll. The Prozac-initiated alertness starts to feel artificial, memory and concentration become impaired, and as one person said to me, "I feel like I'm on some kind of binge."

Prozac was the first widely available drug truly useful for mild to moderate depression.

For this reason, physicians typically start with a different antidepressant, such as Paxil or Serzone, when treating patients with severe insomnia. If they do prescribe Prozac, they may have to prescribe a second drug for use at night. However, for those people in whom depression causes excess sleep, Prozac is often a perfect choice.

Reduced sleeping isn't the only stimulating side effect of Prozac. It can also cause increased daytime agitation and irritability. Some people report a peculiar internal restlessness that makes them fidget incessantly and want to chew gum. Other symptoms include a general increase in anxiety, along with such symptoms as dry mouth, heart palpitations, and hypervigilance. One person said, "I feel like I've had ten cups of coffee when I'm on Prozac."

However, many people feel nothing but a gentle and subtle increase in energy when they take Prozac, and a few even report drowsiness. Others who do experience side effects find that the most unpleasant ones fade away over time. Such variability of results is a phenomenon seen with all drugs and makes a certain amount of individual trial and error unavoidable.

Eileen's Story

Depression itself can interfere with a normal sex life. Eileen wasn't worried about the sexual side effects of Prozac because depression had already taken away her interest in sex. At age 47, it had been almost 10 years since she'd thought of sex with enthusiasm. For her, this was actually the only symptom of depression and the reason why her doctor thought to recommend Prozac.

Four weeks after starting the drug, Eileen was surprised to catch herself feeling sexual again. For a couple of months she and her husband enjoyed a healthy sex life thanks to Prozac. But then came the catch.

"After about 3 months orgasms became difficult, and soon they were impossible. I was in the opposite situation from before. Previously, I didn't care. Now I cared, but hit a brick wall."

Eileen's depression was not severe, and because anorgasmia has not been reported with St. John's wort, it may be an appropriate option for her.

For women, Prozac often causes a different type of side effect: anorgasmia, the inability to experience orgasm. Although sexual arousal may still be possible, orgasm can't be achieved, and these women are left frustrated and unsatisfied.

The official list of Prozac side effects reports anorgasmia as rare, but in clinical practice it is one of the most common reasons patients quit taking the drug. In fact, anorgasmia is so prevalent that at least two competing antidepressants are specifically marketed as not interfering with orgasm (Serzone and Wellbutrin). Possible reasons for this discrepancy will be addressed later in this chapter.

In men, this side effect can manifest as difficulty achieving ejaculation or frank impotence, but such problems are less frequent than female anorgasmia. Some men even appreciate this side effect. They find that Prozac successfully treats premature ejaculation and may take it specifically for that purpose.

Prozac can cause insomnia, agitation, inability to experience orgasm, impotence, headaches, and nausea.

Besides interfering with orgasm, Prozac can also cause a decrease in libido. This side effect occurs in both men and women, and it can be extremely unpleasant. One person said to me, "I like feeling less depressed, but sex just doesn't seem to exist for me anymore. It's like a part of me has been chopped out." Again, this doesn't happen to everyone: For some, Prozac almost seems to act as an aphrodisiac.

Another common side effect of Prozac is headache. According to the official statistics, 20% of people on Prozac develop headaches. This is not quite as problematic as it sounds, however, because 15% of the individuals given placebo in the official studies also developed headaches. The mere thought of taking a drug, it appears, is enough to make one's head hurt.

Nevertheless, the headaches caused by Prozac can be severe, probably more severe than placebo headaches. Several patients of mine developed full-blown migraine attacks for the first time in their lives when they started Prozac, and in a few cases it took a month or two afterward to resolve this problem. However, this is yet another example of the unpredictability of drugs—Prozac actually *prevents* migraines in many people.

Other physical problems caused by Prozac include nausea and diarrhea. According to official statistics, 21.1%

of those who take Prozac develop nausea and 12.3% develop diarrhea, and these numbers appear to coincide fairly well with clinical experience. Weight loss due to loss of appetite may also occur, although seldom dramatically enough to make Prozac an effective diet pill.

Another common complaint of people who take Prozac is that they "can't think straight." I have mentioned how drug-induced sleep deprivation can cause impaired memory and concentration, but Prozac seems to cause these side effects directly in some people. Symptoms include walking into a room and not remembering why ("destinesia," as a friend calls it), forgetting appointments, and being unable to stay on a single train of thought.

> **Zoloft, Paxil, and Luvox all work similarly to Prozac. However, when one member of the Prozac-Zoloft-Paxil-Luvox group fails, another may succeed.**

The most dramatic adverse effects attributed to Prozac concern the specter of increased violence toward self or others. This charge first appeared in 1990, when Dr. Martin Teicher of McLean Hospital reported that six of his depressed patients had suddenly developed intense suicidal tendencies after starting Prozac. Subsequently, several lawsuits were instituted claiming that Prozac had caused violent criminal aggression. Overnight Prozac gained the reputation of being a killer drug.

It is easy to be misled, however, by anecdotal reports. Most of the violent acts attributed to Prozac use were committed by people with a previous history of violence. Did Prozac cause that violence, or was it just a convenient excuse? It's also important to note that suicide is a classic feature of depression itself. Therefore, could it be that what seemed to be a suicide brought on by Prozac was only a suicide Prozac failed to prevent? Since more people were taking Prozac than had ever taken any other antidepressant before, the number of individual cases of suicide while on Prozac would naturally be comparatively higher.

Wellbutrin narrowly missed *being* **Prozac.**

Indeed, careful evaluation of the data showed that, on a percentage basis, people taking Prozac didn't commit suicide any more often than those taking the older antidepressants. Prozac is not actually a murderer.

This piece of information isn't the last word on the subject, however. On average, Prozac probably *reduces* the suicide rate of depressed people, by treating their depression. It is still possible, nonetheless, that Prozac may increase the potential for suicide in *certain* individuals. That is certainly Martin Teicher's impression, and there is no reason to dispute his words. Drugs are frequently known to cause peculiar ("idiosyncratic") effects in a few individuals. Prozac may present a real danger of violence to only a small subset of the population.

A potentially more serious unresolved concern regarding the safety of Prozac is the possibility of long-term side effects. It is far more difficult to establish the safety of a drug over an extended period than to determine immediate adverse consequences. Safety tests for drugs are very seldom carried beyond 8 weeks. If Prozac were to cause side effects after, say, 15 years of use, there is no way to know now; the drug simply hasn't been in use that long.

Actually, for most drugs, long-term risks remain unknown. Problems that take a long time to develop are typically discovered only by accident. But many drugs are taken to prevent relatively serious medical complications. The trade-off of known benefit versus unknown risk may be worth making.

Major depression is a disease that can cause death. Using antidepressants to prevent immediate harm may be worth the risk of unidentified consequences down the road. But Prozac is now being used almost casually. Doctors are prescribing it for a great variety of symptoms—from PMS to premature ejaculation—and the implicit trade-off of short-term benefit versus long-term risk may not be worth it for many of these conditions.

The most widely discussed concern is that Prozac may cause a delayed syndrome similar to *tardive dyskinesia*. This term refers to abnormal movements (dyskinesias) that appear after years, or even decades, of taking antischizophrenic medication (thus they are "tardy" symptoms). The uncontrollable movements of tardive dyskinesia are quite unpleasant, involving lip smacking, tongue rolling, and facial grimacing. The worst part of this syndrome is that it doesn't necessarily go away after discontinuing medication. Tardive dyskinesia is often forever.

There is no guarantee that Prozac won't produce its own syndrome in people who take it for a long time; and there's considerable reason to suspect it might. Although tardive dyskinesia isn't understood completely, it seems to be a kind of permanent version of typical antischizophrenic side effects. What if the excessively energizing effects of Prozac could become permanent, too, leading to a syndrome of unrelenting agitation, restlessness, and insomnia? Purely speculation at this point; but considering the history of disastrous side effects caused by other drugs, perhaps it should be taken seriously.

Whatever its long-term implications, Prozac has shown remarkably low immediate toxicity. Individuals who have attempted to commit suicide while taking Prozac have generally experienced only relatively mild symptoms from overdose, such as vomiting and agitation, although seizures have also occurred in rare instances.

Why Does the Official List of Prozac's Side Effects Look So Good?

Despite the problems previously described, the official statistics on Prozac's side effects show a drug that seems to be almost side-effect–free. The *Physicians' Desk Reference (PDR)* lists an incidence of sexual side effects, for example, that is under 2%. This seems to be so different from the clinical experience of practitioners that there has to be an explanation. And there is.

The initial studies on Prozac lasted for only 4 to 6 weeks. Anorgasmia often takes somewhat longer than that to develop, and even if it did occur in that interval, women might not immediately connect the symptom with the drug. Thus, to detect anorgasmia, the screening period was simply too short.

Furthermore, special interviewing techniques are essential for eliciting accurate reports on sensitive subjects, such as sexual dysfunction. Many people may simply not be willing to admit such problems. Studies performed by researchers experienced in the field of sexual dysfunction have shown substantially higher rates of such problems in people taking antidepressants, perhaps as high as 1 in 3.[1]

How Well Does Prozac Actually Work for Depression?

How well does Prozac work for depression? The answer to this fundamental question remains surprisingly unclear, not only for Prozac but for all antidepressants. Depression is not easy to evaluate scientifically. Unlike high blood pressure or diabetes, the extent of a person's depression can't be measured by a machine. Depression is primarily a subjective experience, and there is no way to get around depending on each individual's own report and each physician's personal impression. Difficult to duplicate and susceptible to the influence of suggestion, these reports and impressions are highly variable.

In order to achieve some sort of objectivity, experimenters use a special interview technique called the Hamilton Depression rating scale (HAM-D). Administered by a physician, the HAM-D is a test that takes into account physical signs, such as slowed speech and movement, as well as answers to questions, such as "Do you frequently cry for no reason?" and "Do you feel fatigued?" Each observation and answer is turned into a number, and a total HAM-D score is created by combining all these numbers. Higher numbers indicate greater depression.

If too high a dose is taken at one time, or if Wellbutrin is combined with certain other drugs, the risk of seizure can reach almost 4%.

The HAM-D interview and others like it are widely used in studies evaluating the effectiveness of antidepressant drugs. In a typical clinical trial, some participants are given placebo, and others a real drug. The HAM-D test is then administered at intervals, and the resulting numbers are compared to evaluate effects on depression of drug and placebo.

Unfortunately, while the HAM-D is much more reliable than simply asking doctors to decide whether individuals seem to improve or not, the scale still leaves a lot to be desired. There is still a lot of subjectivity involved. When various physicians administer the HAM-D to a single person, they may come up with different results. For best results it is recommended that all the physicians involved in a study learn the use of the HAM-D from a sin-

The Power of Placebo

Just how powerful is placebo treatment? Very powerful. In most studies, up to 30% of participants show dramatic improvement with placebo pills, and for certain illnesses this reaches as high as 50%. Placebo pills also cause a high incidence of imaginary side effects. This is why double-blind studies are so important. Yet medical researchers in America seem to have overlooked the possibility that drugs with a high incidence of side effects may break the blind.

In Europe, researchers take this problem much more seriously. They frequently ask participants in such studies to guess whether they are getting a real drug or placebo. If many more than 50% guess right, researchers rethink the whole experiment.

Psychologists Roger Greenburg and Seymour Fisher further explore the magnitude of this effect in an article that attempts to evaluate the true effectiveness of Prozac and other antidepressants.[2] They suggest that all double-blind trials need to take into account the side effects of drugs and their influence on results.

With Prozac, one method to get around this problem might be to use caffeine pills as placebos instead of sugar pills. Then at least both groups would feel a stimulant effect. However, this has never been tried. We are therefore in the position of not really knowing how well Prozac works with the placebo effect subtracted.

gle teacher in order to make their rating styles similar. But this step is often skipped, and even when it is followed, the results remain far from consistent. Different doctors' assessments may still differ widely, and, as shown in the following text, there is plenty of room for the influence of suggestion.

Limitations in the reliability of HAM-D aren't the only obstacles to obtaining reliable estimates of Prozac's effectiveness. A potentially more serious problem lies in the nature of controlled experiments themselves.

In a proper double-blind study, neither the doctor nor the participant can tell the difference between placebo and drug. In other words, they are both "blind" in order to prevent the power of suggestion from skewing the results.

When antidepressants cause side effects such as drowsiness, fainting, sexual dysfunction, and weight gain, it's hard to tell that you're not depressed.

When people know they are taking a real drug, they have a strong inclination to expect results, which may actually produce them. The reverse naturally occurs for placebos. Similarly, a doctor aware of what is in a capsule may inadvertently communicate positive or negative suggestion by body language or tone of voice. To keep a test unbiased, it is essential that there is no way to tell placebo and real medication apart. They are usually packaged identically, and their identity is kept secret from all but a committee overseeing the experiment.

Because Prozac causes a significant number of side effects, however, individuals taking Prozac may be perfectly aware that what they are getting isn't placebo. The difference may be as immediately apparent to them as that between caffeinated coffee and decaf. Thus a seemingly double-blind experiment could in fact be perfectly transparent.

This loss of blinding means that the power of suggestion can creep in, and the power of suggestion should never be underestimated. Years of experience have shown that positive expectation has the power to improve almost all diseases. Considering all the media hype surrounding Prozac, its suggestive power may be very great indeed.

Individuals who believe they are taking an effective drug are inclined to take an optimistic view of their symptoms and typically persuade themselves to believe that they're feeling better. This can lead to improved HAM-D scores. But placebo can do more than that; it can actually speed up recovery. This is known to be the case for many illnesses, including such objective ones as infections; and when the disease is already a psychological one, psychological influences are undoubtedly even stronger. Depressed individuals who know they are being given Prozac may say to themselves, "Since I'm taking a powerful drug, I'm going to be less depressed soon." This will create a kind of positive self-talk that can be as beneficial as expensive psychotherapy.

Furthermore, Prozac's particular side effects may enhance the drug's placebo potential because these effects relate specifically to the disease being treated. Stimulant effects simulate relief from depression, which may convince people that their depression is lifting, providing their imaginations with more fodder for positive thinking. There's nothing wrong with positive suggestion, of course. However, it can obscure determining the effectiveness of Prozac per se.

Just like their patients, physicians have implicit faith in the power of drugs, too—especially new drugs. This faith might distort the outcome of Prozac-placebo comparison experiments in the following manner: By observing increased fidgeting or from the patient's reports of increased insomnia, a doctor administering the HAM-D may come to suspect that a particular individual is taking Prozac rather than placebo. This suspicion may be conscious or unconscious. In either case, when administering the HAM-D, the doctor may inadvertently skew his or her observations to reflect expectation of improvement.

I'm not suggesting that the studies are completely wrong and that Prozac is a fake. The medication obviously works. But just how much its real effects are amplified by suggestion remains unclear. This same problem applies to all other antidepressants. St. John's wort, on the other hand, doesn't appear to cause side effects. As I will describe later, this actually may prove a handicap against the herb in scientific studies, by depriving it of a similar placebo power.

Zoloft, Paxil, and Luvox: Three Alternatives to Prozac

Zoloft, Paxil, and Luvox work similarly to Prozac. However, while these medications also inhibit serotonin reuptake, they are chemically distinct and sometimes produce different clinical effects. It is not rare to find that when one member of the Prozac-Zoloft-Paxil-Luvox group fails, another may succeed.

On average, none of the drugs in this group has been shown to be better than another with regard to efficacy or the extent of side effects. But some *individuals* do better with one than another. The situation is similar to what is commonly seen in results from the many anti-inflammatory pills used for pain. Overall, they're pretty similar, but certain people respond best to a particular drug from among that family of drugs.

A dramatic example of this phenomenon occurred one day in my private practice: Two individuals who didn't know each other came in one right after the other. They both were complaining of pain from a sprained ankle. The first one told me she had tried Naprosyn without luck, but when she switched to ibuprofen, she immediately felt better. The other person told me exactly the reverse of that story. Individual variation of this type is completely normal, and the advantage of having a variety of drugs to choose from is that if one doesn't work well there are other options.

Generally, Paxil tends to be the least stimulating of the three drugs. It actually causes tiredness in a significant number of individuals who take it. This may make it preferable to Prozac for those who suffer from anxiety and insomnia, and less useful for those who complain of fatigue and excessive sleep. Luvox and Zoloft stand somewhere in the middle, while Prozac is the most energizing. But these are only average effects, and some people experience them completely differently.

The same is true of other side effects. While the overall frequency of headaches, nausea, and confusion seems to be roughly similar among these

The MAO inhibitors are among the few medications with which you must watch what you eat to avoid deadly reactions. Dangerous foods include cheese, dried meat, dried fish, canned figs, broad beans, and concentrated yeast products, as well as vermouth and other wines.

drugs, certain patients may develop particular side effects in response to one drug and not another. However, sexual side effects seem to be more uniform. If a particular person experiences these with one SSRI, he or she will most likely have the same problem with the other ones too.

Trazodone and Serzone: May Help Insomnia, Too

Trazodone is one of the first serotonin-specific drugs developed, although it isn't an SSRI and doesn't raise serotonin levels as dramatically as Prozac. The biggest problem with trazodone is that it causes a great deal of drowsiness. Because of this powerful side effect, trazodone has come to be used more widely as a sleeping pill than as an antidepressant. It is one of the drugs commonly given in combination with stimulating antidepressants to counteract drug-induced insomnia.

Serzone is known unofficially as "son of trazodone," and it isn't usually classified as an SSRI either. Its particular claim to fame is that (unlike the SSRIs) it doesn't seem to cause a high incidence of sexual dysfunction. In advertising, the pharmaceutical representatives often heavily emphasize this characteristic, offering Serzone as a substitute antidepressant for people who can't tolerate Prozac.

However, Serzone has thus far failed to make a major impact. It causes less drowsiness than trazodone, but its effect still tends toward somnolence. As one person described it, "When I'm on Serzone I feel like I'm swimming through soup." Serzone is useful primarily for those in whom anxiety and insomnia are a significant component of depression.

Wellbutrin: Just Missed *Being* Prozac

Wellbutrin narrowly missed *being* Prozac. It was approved as an antidepressant in 1985, two years before Prozac's release, and if it weren't for early reports of increased seizure activity in those using it, Peter Kramer's book would probably have been called *Listening to Wellbutrin.*

Although it was eventually discovered that Wellbutrin could be safe when used correctly, its reputation was tainted and its release delayed. Prozac was already firmly established as the dominant antidepressant by the time Wellbutrin came back into circulation.

Many physicians remain leery of prescribing Wellbutrin out of fear of causing seizures. If too high a dose is taken at one time, or if Wellbutrin is combined with certain other drugs, the risk of seizure can reach almost 4%. Nonetheless, Wellbutrin is a useful medication when used carefully. Its great advantage is that, although it is fully as energizing as Prozac, it doesn't cause sexual dysfunction. Like Prozac, Wellbutrin can cause insomnia, agitation, restlessness, and anxiety, as well as nausea, headache, and dry mouth.

The mechanism of action in Wellbutrin remains unknown. It produces no significant effect on norepinephrine or serotonin and only weakly increases levels of the biological amine dopamine, thus confounding the amine hypothesis. Wellbutrin proves that we don't understand the biological basis of depression.

Effexor: When SSRIs Fail

Although Prozac's original claim to fame was that its action was specific, with Effexor we come full circle. Its manufacturer has advertised the fact that it raises both norepinephrine and serotonin levels. Unlike tricyclic antidepressants that do the same thing, however, Effexor usually produces an energizing effect.

Effexor is frequently tried when SSRIs fail. It typically produces a higher incidence of some side effects than the Prozac-Paxil-Zoloft-Luvox group, particularly nausea, but it doesn't seem to impair orgasm as often as the SSRIs. Otherwise, the side effects are rather similar.

Tricyclics: Not for Mild to Moderate Depression

Prior to the release of Prozac, the most widely used family of antidepressants belonged to this category. The name comes from the three circular chemical structures found in the tricyclic molecule. Imipramine was the first tricyclic antidepressant, and subsequent drugs in the family all bear striking similarities. Some of the more famous are Elavil (amitriptyline), Sinequan (doxepin), and Pamelor (nortriptyline).

All of these antidepressants have demonstrable and equivalent effectiveness in the treatment of major depression. Nevertheless, they cause too many side effects to be useful in the treatment of mild to moderate depression. The tricyclics were originally derived from antihistamines, and they still carry the entire list of classic side effects associated with antihistamines, such as drowsiness, blurred vision, dry mouth, constipation, sweating, heart palpitations, weight gain, dizziness, and urinary retention. Sometimes these side effects can be even greater in the antidepressants than the antihistamines because of the high dosages necessary to produce full antidepressant benefits.

Recently, antihistamines have been developed that are relatively side-effect–free, such as Claritin, principally because they can't get into the brain to produce drowsiness. But tricyclics *must* get into the brain to produce their antidepressant effects, allowing the full range of symptoms to occur. Most tricyclic antidepressants make excellent sleeping pills. (And most of them are pretty decent antihistamines, as well!) Other common side effects include fainting, sexual dysfunction, and weight gain.

With side effects like these, it's hard to tell you're not depressed. Drowsiness, dry mouth, and weight gain may be a reasonable price to pay for relief from major depression. But for mild to moderate depression, the side effects of these older antidepressants are often worse than the disease—and depressing in their own right.

In *Listening to Prozac,* Peter Kramer speculates for many pages on why Prozac took off in a way the tricyclic antidepressants never did. He wonders whether Prozac "touches features of depression" Pamelor can't reach, and hypothesizes that serotonin may be more fundamentally related to depression than the amines raised by tricyclics (primarily norepinephrine). But there is a simpler explanation that is more likely: side effects.

Considering all the side effects of drugs, St. John's wort might be an even better choice for mild to moderate depression.

Pamelor causes more side effects than Prozac, and the ones it causes are precisely the ones you don't want if you suffer from mild to moderate depression. Prozac's immediate stimulation creates a positive suggestion of recovery from depression, while Pamelor's drowsiness connotes deepening illness. Thus both the side effects of tricyclics and the suggestions that they provide to the imagination are exactly wrong. Tricyclics simply aren't good drugs for treatment of mild to moderate depression.

MAO Inhibitors: Powerful but Dangerous

This is the oldest category of antidepressants, and if it weren't for the known risks they pose, the MAO inhibitors would be much more widely used. Representative drugs include Marplan (isocarboxazid), Nardil (phenylzine), and Parnate (tranylcypromine).

Drugs in this family poison the enzyme called *monoamine-oxidase.* Monoamine-oxidase is a "garbage cleaner" enzyme in charge of breaking down excess biological amines. When monoamine-oxidase is poisoned, the levels of numerous brain chemicals, including amines, begin to rise. As you'll recall, low amine levels are believed to be one of the causes of depression. The MAO inhibitors are some of the most powerful antidepressants known, perhaps because of their wide spectrum of action. They are energizing and can produce dramatic reductions in symptoms. Unfortunately, they cause many side effects and can even cause death if not used with extreme care.

The dangers of these drugs come directly from the way they work. The job of the MAO-scavenger enzyme is to control the levels of biological amines. When a person takes an MAO inhibitor, the amine levels naturally begin to rise. The goal is to raise them just enough to help combat depression. However, there's a fine line between just enough and too much. If the levels of biological amines pass a certain threshold, they begin to cause extremely high blood pressure and the risk of death by brain hemorrhage.

The usual cause of this is additional amines taken by mouth. Numerous other drugs contain amines, such as Ritalin, ephedrine, pseudoephedrine (Sudafed), phenylpropanolamine (also found in over-the-counter cold and allergy remedies), and asthma medications. A person on MAO inhibitors must avoid these medications religiously. (Prozac, tricyclic antidepressants, insulin, oral diabetes drugs, and Antabuse can also cause serious reactions in someone taking an MAO inhibitor, but by somewhat different mechanisms.)

Drugs aren't the only problem. The MAO inhibitors are among the few medications with which you must watch what you eat. A substance called tyramine occurs in many foods, and it is a natural relative of the body's biologically active amines. If a tyramine-containing food is consumed by a person taking an MAO inhibitor, this may be enough to trigger a fatal reaction. Dangerous foods include cheese, dried meat, dried fish, canned figs, broad beans, and concentrated yeast products, as well as vermouth and other wines. People taking MAO inhibitors must treat these common foods as deadly poisons.

Because of this unique risk and the dietary challenge it presents, MAO inhibitors are only rarely used today. However, they are still tried sometimes when all else fails.

Beyond Drugs: Psychotherapy

Although drug therapy is rapidly becoming the mainstay of conventional treatment for depression, it isn't the only accepted approach. Conventional medicine still accepts the benefit of psychotherapy (although sometimes grudgingly, because treatment of psychological disorders simply doesn't fit the medical model very well). Medical doctors are usually much more comfortable prescribing drugs.

One problem plaguing psychotherapy's acceptance is that its effectiveness is next to impossible to evaluate scientifically. Double-blind experiments are difficult even to conceive. Nonetheless, the research that has been performed seems to indicate that psychotherapy can be an effective treatment for depression.

One great advantage of psychotherapy is that, unlike drugs, it can produce positive effects that "belong to you." These benefits continue long after therapy stops and may enrich the rest of your life. The same can't be said of any drug, nor of St. John's wort. But psychotherapy is expensive, time consuming, and not always successful. Should psychotherapy not work fully, or if it simply isn't an option, taking an antidepressant drug may prove useful. Considering all the side effects of drugs, St. John's wort might be an even better choice for mild to moderate depression. From the chapter that follows, you will learn how to treat depression with this safe, natural, and essentially side-effect–free herb.

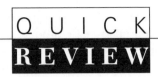

- There are many types of antidepressants. Although all are equally effective in treating severe major depression, the newer drugs are more appropriate for mild to moderate depression because they cause less fatigue. Side effects, however, are still a problem.

- The most common side effects with Prozac are nausea, insomnia, headache, and sexual difficulties. Zoloft, Paxil, and Effexor produce similar side effects. Wellbutrin does not cause sexual problems but it can cause seizures.

- Serzone and trazadone are not very useful for mild to moderate depression because they tend to produce severe fatigue.

- Drugs in the tricyclic category typically cause fatigue, dry mouth, and other unpleasant symptoms.

- MAO inhibitors can cause dangerous reactions when combined with certain foods or drugs.

CHAPTER

FIVE

St. John's Wort

The Scientific Evidence

Alternative medicine includes many unproven and worthless treatments. However, St. John's wort does not fall into either of these categories. Both its effectiveness and its side effects have received significant scientific evaluation. This chapter describes the results of the best St. John's wort research, as well as the experience of clinicians who use it.

What Research Says About St. John's Wort's Effectiveness

According to a report in the August 1996 edition of the *British Medical Journal,* there have now been 23 randomized double-blind clinical trials of St. John's wort in the treatment of depression.[1] The total number of participants involved in these studies has reached a respectable 1,757, presenting a compelling case for this traditional herbal treatment. For comparison, a typical total number of participants for drug validation trials is between 1,000 and 2,000.[2] However, not all of the St. John's wort studies were of the highest quality.

Some studies compared St. John's wort against placebo, while others compared St. John's wort against a pharmaceutical antidepressant. This chapter covers comparisons between St. John's wort and placebo, leaving the herb-drug comparisons for chapter 8.

The total number of patients involved in St. John's wort studies has reached a respectable 1,757, presenting a compelling case for this traditional herbal treatment.

One of the best designed studies was a 4-week comparison of St. John's wort and placebo performed in 1993 by the German physician K. D. Hansgen and his colleagues.[3] In this study 72 participants from 11 different physicians' practices were selected based on standard *Diagnostic Statistical Manual of Mental Disorders (DSM)* criteria for major depression. (More people were later added to the study.) The study design followed the standard research design used to validate phar- maceutical antidepressants.

In order to measure the extent of improvement produced by St. John's wort, Hansgen used the HAM-D rating scale for depression. As you may recall from my earlier explanation, the HAM-D combines physicians' observations and individuals' answers to questions in order to yield a number that represents the severity of depression. Higher numbers indicate more serious depression and lower numbers indicate milder depression.

At the beginning of this study, participants were rated according to the HAM-D to determine the starting levels

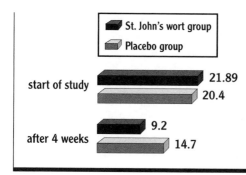

Figure 2. *Ham-D scores after 4 weeks in a double-blind study (Higher scores indicate greater depression.)* (Hansgen, 1993)

of their depression. Then half the participants were given a standard dose of St. John's wort, the other half placebo. At 2 and 4 weeks, the individuals were retested and their scores recorded (see figure 2).

Those taking St. John's wort showed significant improvement. Their HAM-D scores dropped from an average of 21.89 prior to treatment to 9.2 after 4 weeks of treatment. This drop of almost 60% compares quite favorably to what is usually seen with antidepressant medication.

As always happens (although it never ceases to surprise), those taking placebo also improved. However, their average HAM-D score only dropped by about 30%, from an initial average of 20.4 to 14.7. Statistically, this difference in results was significant.

Another way of looking at this data is that 81% of the participants taking St. John's wort improved significantly (greater than a 50% drop in their scores), while only 26% of the placebo group responded. Again, this was a statistically significant result.

Three participants on placebo dropped out of the study because their symptoms of depression became too severe to continue. This did not happen in the St. John's wort group.

The psychiatrists involved in the study also used two other methods of measuring levels of depression to con-

firm the HAM-D results, and these gave substantially the same result. Overall, the difference in outcomes between individuals on placebo and those on St. John's wort easily exceeded the requirements for statistical significance.

Unfortunately, the NIH has chosen to study the effectiveness of St. John's wort in moderate to severe depression rather than mild to moderate depression.

During the course of this study, only one person taking St. John's wort reported any adverse effect (disturbance in sleep), while two people on placebo said they developed stomach upset.

The scientific quality of this study was reasonably good. Its method of randomization followed standard guidelines, the techniques of statistical analysis used were mathematically acceptable, study dropouts were accounted for, adverse reactions were indicated, and the double-blind method was preserved throughout.

In one sense, at least, this study was superior to typical antidepressant versus placebo trials. Drugs cause side effects; and, as I pointed out in the preceding chapter, those effects may allow participants to distinguish between drug and placebo, even when they look exactly alike. Thus the influence of the power of suggestion cannot be excluded from drug versus placebo tests. This makes the legitimacy of all double-blind studies for traditional antidepressant medication somewhat suspect. However, no similar problem occurs with the essentially side-effect–free St. John's wort.

While this multicenter study makes a compelling case for St. John's wort, a total of 72 participants (minus dropouts) is not enough by itself to establish the effectiveness of a treatment. Therefore, an additional 36 patients were added to the trial in 1996, and the study methodology was repeated.[4] The results followed exactly the same pattern as before.

The Hansgen study involved individuals whose depression was moderately severe. (They suffered from major depression, but only moderately severe major depression. As mentioned in chapter 2, the language is definitely confusing!) In severe major depression, HAM-D scores are 25 or higher, while in this study the participants averaged less than 22. In a separate study, the effectiveness of St. John's wort was evaluated for mildly depressed patients (with an average HAM-D of about 16). The 105 participants were drawn from 3 physicians' practices and followed for 4 weeks.[5] At the end of the study, 67% of those on St. John's wort showed satisfactory response to treatment (a greater than 50% reduction in their HAM-D scores), compared to only 28% of those individuals on placebo. Significant improvements were particularly noted in mood, anxiety, and insomnia.

One of the longest studies on St. John's wort was performed in 1991. It followed 50 participants for 8 weeks, and once more the herb proved significantly more effective than placebo.[6] Yet another multicenter study, performed in 1991, showed positive results in 116 individuals followed for 6 weeks.[7] This study suffered, however, from one significant drawback: The St. John's wort was administered in the form of drops, which may have been distinguishable by taste from placebo.

A recent study looked at the effectiveness of a new kind of St. John's wort extract standardized to its content of a substance called hyperforin, rather than to hypericin[8] (see chapter 6 for more information on standardized extracts). It was designed to test the theory that hyperforin may be an active ingredient in St. John's wort. However, it also supplies additional evidence that the herb is an effective treatment for depression.

Recent research suggests that St. John's wort may work by raising serotonin levels.

For a period of 42 days, 147 people diagnosed with mild to moderate depression according to the *DSM-IV* (the most modern psychiatric diagnostic guide) were given either placebo or one of two forms of St. John's wort: a low hyperforin product (0.5%) or a high hyperforin product (5%). As usual, the HAM-D was used to determine improvement.

The results showed that the form of St. John's wort containing 5% hyperforin was successful in controlling symptoms of depression in about 50% of cases, a better result than placebo and only a little lower than what has been seen in other trials of St. John's wort. However, the low hyperforin product did not do any better than placebo.

We will return to the question of whether hyperforin is the active ingredient in St. John's wort later in this chapter.

In 1995 E. Ernst published a formal review of the literature, ranking the trials based on standard scientific criteria and eliminating those with significant flaws.[9] Out of the 14 studies that compared St. John's wort against placebo, Ernst narrowed the field to 9 studies involving over 600 participants. All of these studies found St. John's wort to be an effective antidepressant. (Ernst did find 2 studies that failed to find a significant effect with St. John's wort, but they were too poorly designed to be included in the review.)

The cumulative results of these carefully selected trials were impressive. Ernst reported that "taken together, these data are scientifically compelling and leave little doubt as to the efficacy of *Hypericum* [St. John's wort] in the treatment of depressive symptoms."

A similar review published in the August 1996 *British Medical Journal* arrived at essentially the same conclusions.[10]

This body of research has been criticized because none of the studies lasted longer than 8 weeks.[11] While this is a valid point, the same criticism applies to most drugs on their initial approval. For example, in the 1997 *Physicians' Desk Reference,* the manufacturer of Prozac states that "the effectiveness of Prozac in long-term use, that is, for more than 5 to 6 weeks, has not been systematically evaluated in controlled trials."[12] In light of this, the St. John's wort evidence certainly deserves to be taken seriously. On this U.S. researchers agree. In 1997 the National Institutes of Health (NIH) announced that it would begin a long-term study comparing the effects of St. John's wort, Zoloft, and placebo. The results of this study (not yet available at the time of this writing) will undoubtedly make a significant impact.

How Does St. John's Wort Work?

As explained in chapter 4, science doesn't really understand how pharmaceutical antidepressants produce their effects. The prevailing theory is that low levels of biological amines (such as serotonin and norepinephrine) can cause depression and that antidepressants function by raising those levels. However, there are many problems with this "amine hypothesis," not the least of which is that some antidepressants function perfectly well without significantly changing the level of any biological amines.

A New Drug?

Presuming that St. John's wort does well in the NIH study, is it possible that it could become an approved drug? There are still two major obstacles.

In order to get a new drug approved, it is necessary to get through many hurdles set by the FDA. The purpose of these hurdles is to prevent dangerous or worthless drugs from entering the market. However, all the necessary reports and studies are very expensive, often exceeding $200 million.

Drug companies gladly pay this expense when they've invented a new drug, because they will own the patent and can earn the money back. But St. John's wort isn't patentable. It's in the public domain as a natural herb. For this reason there isn't any obvious source of the necessary funds to get it approved.

Therefore, the amine hypothesis must be only part of the story. Nonetheless, it's the only explanation we have thus far. For this reason researchers have investigated whether St. John's wort changes amine levels, too. At this point, the results remain inconclusive.

Early research seemed to indicate that extracts of St. John's wort inhibit the enzyme monoamine-oxidase.[13] This indication placed the herb in the MAO-inhibitor class of antidepressants and spawned a series of warnings about not eating certain foods while taking it. However, these studies involved applying extracts of St. John's wort directly into test tubes. Later investigation showed that the dosages of St. John's wort taken orally in actual practice are probably 100 times too low to inhibit monoamine-oxidase.[14] MAO inhibition is no longer considered a likely explanation for St. John's wort's effectiveness in treating depression.

Another problem is that batches of herbs are not inter-changeable. As described further in chapter 6, a drug is a drug, but each St. John's wort plant is a little different from every other. Details of weather, soil, time of picking, and numerous other factors can effect potency. Even if one batch was proven to work for depression, how would we know that the next year's crop could do the same? The FDA is not likely to approve a product that might work some years and not others.

More likely, standardized extracts of St. John's wort might become approved over-the-counter drugs, where the regulation is less stringent. Other herbs such as cascara sagrada (a laxative) have been approved in this way.

More recent research suggests that St. John's wort may actually function like the SSRIs by inhibiting the reuptake of serotonin. In one study, researchers added St. John's wort to test tubes filled with primeval nerve cells and observed that serotonin receptors seemed to be suppressed.[15] They theorized that the herb might therefore function by impairing the reuptake of serotonin into cells.

This highly theoretical study did not, however, investigate whether normal dosages of St. John's wort can raise serotonin levels. Another study attempted to answer this practical question by examining the brains of rats and mice who were fed St. John's wort extracts.[16] Serotonin and dopamine levels did rise significantly in treated animals. Nevertheless, this experiment produced a surprising finding: A preparation of St. John's wort in which the hypericin was removed still caused the same effect. Another animal study showed that St. John's wort inhibited reuptake of serotonin, dopamine, and norepinephrine.[17]

Recent evidence suggests that a different ingredient of St. John's wort called hyperforin, may be the active antidepressant substance in the herb. Besides the double-blind trial discussed earlier in this chapter, unpublished evidence was presented at a major conference in March of 1998 further suggesting that it is hyperforin and not hypericin that matters.[18] However, these findings have been disputed, and further research will be necessary to resolve the matter.

What does this all mean? Well, because these studies are preliminary, it is fair to say that, at this point, we really do not know how St. John's wort works in treating depression. However, this only puts St. John's wort in the good company of other antidepressants, whose precise method of function remains unclear, as well. With St. John's wort there is one further level of mystery. As for many herbs, its active ingredients are not known. Most likely, numerous substances work together to produce the antidepressant effect.

What Doctors Say

An increasing number of U.S. physicians have begun to experiment with St. John's wort in recent years. Their clinical impressions confirm the results of published literature and paint a picture of a treatment that is substantially effective in real life.

One such physician is Scott Shannon, a psychiatrist in Fort Collins, Colorado. Dr. Shannon was a student of Dr. Andrew Weil and has spent much of his professional career exploring alternative options for emotional illness. In Shannon's opinion, St. John's wort is often effective in mild to moderate depression. "It elevates mood and raises energy, without causing side effects," he says. "Patients tell me they feel brighter, less fatigued, and more able to manage."

He tells the story of Karol, a woman in her mid-50s, who was burdened by numerous responsibilities. "She had lots of irons in the fire," Shannon says. "Young children, aging parents, work stresses—it was all a bit too much for her. She felt chronically depressed and anxious."

Karol tried Paxil, and although she found it helpful, she couldn't tolerate the sexual side effects. Shannon switched her to St. John's wort, and she responded within a few weeks. "She started to wake up with a sense of liveliness she hadn't felt for a while," he explains. "During the day, she felt less glum and had more energy. She also found it easier to manage stress."

Furthermore, all these benefits occurred without side effects. "She tolerated the St. John's wort without any problems," Shannon says. "I very seldom see any side effects with St. John's wort, other than occasional mild stomach irritation."

We don't really know how St. John's wort works in treating depression. However, this only puts St. John's wort in the good company of other antidepressants.

Besides increased energy and improved mood, my own patients sometimes report normalized appetite, improved sleep, decreased anxiety, reduction in chronic pain, and an increased sense of self-esteem when they start St. John's wort. "When you feel better overall," Shannon says, "it's natural for other symptoms to improve."

Like other clinicians who use St. John's wort, Shannon feels the herb is most appropriate for mild to moderate depression. "St. John's wort is basically a mood elevator and [an] energizer," he says. "It's often my first choice for mild depression because it works well without side effects. However," he cautions, "it isn't appropriate for severe major depression, especially if there's a risk of suicide. Drug treatment is better for major depression. Drugs are also better for people with severe and complex psychological trauma, and when there are vegetative signs."

Vegetative signs are the physical symptoms that often accompany major depression, such as slowed speech and movement. These symptoms generally indicate a more severe form of depression, probably too severe for St. John's wort.

Are drugs always more powerful than St. John's wort? "Usually," says Shannon, "although they cause more side effects, as well." But there can be surprises. Jacqueline Fields, a family practitioner in Loveland, Colorado, tells the story of an elderly man in a nursing home who actually did better on St. John's wort than on antidepressant medication.

"Bruce was too depressed to eat well or talk very much to other patients," she says. "He would just lie around most of the time sleeping. We gave him Zoloft, but it didn't seem to do any good. However, when we started him on St. John's wort, the results were pretty impressive. He got out of bed, ate better, and actually started talking with the other residents."

This story almost sounds like an example of St. John's wort successfully treating severe, major depression. But such a high level of effectiveness seems to be unusual. Most clinicians I've interviewed feel that St. John's wort is typically not as potent as drug treatment. It seldom treats severe depression successfully, and even for mild to moderate depression, medications such as Prozac appear to be somewhat more powerful. St. John's wort's side-effect profile is so superior, however, that for many cases of mild to moderate depression, it may be the best option.

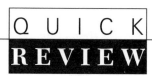

- Strong scientific evidence tells us that St. John's wort is an effective treatment for mild to moderate depression.
- According to good double-blind studies, St. John's wort produces marked improvements in the symptoms of depression over a period of approximately 4 weeks.
- We do not know precisely how St. John's wort works. Current evidence suggests that it is not an MAO inhibitor (as previously thought) but rather affects serotonin levels.
- Clinicians who prescribe St. John's wort feel that the herb is generally somewhat less effective than drug treatment, but may be preferable because it produces far fewer side effects.

How to Take St. John's Wort

After learning about the benefits of St. John's wort, you are probably ready to know how to take it. The subject is a bit more complicated than it sounds, however, because St. John's wort is an herb instead of a drug; and certain concerns regarding standardization must be explained before I can sensibly provide the appropriate dosage.

When you purchase a drug, you generally know exactly what you are getting. Drugs are single chemicals that can be measured and quantified down to their molecular structure. Thus a tablet of extra-strength Tylenol contains 500 mg of acetaminophen, no matter where or when you buy it.

But herbs are living organisms comprised of thousands of ingredients, and between one plant and another the proportions of all these ingredients may be dramatically different. Numerous influences can affect the nature of a given crop. Whether it was grown at the top or bottom of a hill, what the weather was like, when it was picked, what other plants lived nearby, and what kind of soil predominated are only a few of the factors that can affect the chemical make-up of an herb.

This is one very important reason medical doctors prefer drugs to whole herbs. Conventional medicine tries to deal in standardized, reproducible methods, but with herbs it is difficult to know exactly what you're dealing with.

To get around this problem, modern herbalists often use what is known as a "standardized herbal extract." This is a concentrated form of an herb, dissolved in alcohol and water, and "boiled down" until a certain fixed percentage of one or more ingredients is reached. For St. John's wort, chemists deliberately achieve a fixed proportion of the substance hypericin: 0.3%, to be precise. Such standardization allows a reasonable degree of reproducibility from batch to batch.

The proper adult dose of St. John's wort: 300 mg 3 times a day.

This is not to say that hypericin is the only active ingredient in St. John's wort. In fact, we're not even certain that it's *one of* the active ingredients. It is only used as a handle in standardized extracts to roughly gauge overall strength. The rest of the herb's ingredients are still included, and are undoubtedly necessary for effectiveness.

This method of standardization isn't perfect. It is still possible that two batches of extract standardized to 0.3% hypericin may differ substantially in the levels of other important constituents. Thus one bottle of standardized St. John's wort may still be better than another.

The potential for differences between standardized products is especially high when varying methods of extraction are used. Virtually all the scientific studies of St. John's wort involved European products that are made using a specific mixture of methanol and water as the extracting fluid. Furthermore, the extraction process was conducted in darkness and at certain specified temperatures.[1] Products extracted by other methods may contain utterly different constituents, even if they are standardized to hypericin content. Fortunately, many U.S. manufacturers are deliberately imitating the European extractive process.

Recently, a new kid has arrived on the block: hyperforin. As described in the last chapter, both published and unpublished studies seem to indicate that this constituent of St. John's wort may be more relevant than hypericin as a basis for creating standardized extracts. More research is necessary to fully decide this issue.

Dosage

Having explained the complexities of formulating and using standardized herbal extracts, I can now describe the proper adult dose of St. John's wort: It is 300 mg 3 times a day of an extract standardized to contain 0.3% hypericin. Based on late-breaking information, new St. John's wort products are arriving on the market that are standardized to 3 to 5% hyperforin. The dose is still 300 mg 3 times daily. Some physicians prefer to prescribe 600 mg in the morning and 300 mg at lunch time, or even 500 mg twice a day. Higher doses are not believed to produce greater benefit. Due to the occasional side effect of stomach irritation, St. John's wort should be taken with food.

Finally, several commercial preparations combine St. John's wort with other natural substances believed effective for depression (see chapter 9). Although there is nothing necessarily wrong with such an approach, I generally prefer targeted treatments to shotgun methods. You simply won't know what is working if you take a pill that contains nine ingredients. Furthermore, combination treatments frequently contain less than optimal dosages of each individual substance.

Dosages for children are discussed in the next chapter.

What to Expect from Treatment

Although every person is different, St. John's wort seems to commonly produce a gentle, gradual elimination of many of the symptoms of mild to moderate depression. However, the nature of these benefits is not fully captured by the rigid language of medical terms. Actual descriptions by people who have found St. John's wort useful may communicate the experience more effectively. However, please remember that anecdotes such as these don't prove anything about St. John's wort. For proof, one must turn to scientific studies, such as those described in chapter 8.

One of the most common statements I hear is that people feel energized and revivified, but without speediness or jaggedness. As one young woman said, "It's more like the energy of a good night's sleep than a cup of coffee."

However, this increase of energy occurs so smoothly you may not be able to notice it right away. Some people only recognize that they've been feeling more energetic when they stop taking St. John's wort and subsequently sink back to their former state of fatigue.

"I had forgotten what it was like," a 37-year-old man said 3 weeks after quitting the herb. "I didn't think it was working at all, but once the St. John's wort wore off, I started to sleepwalk through my day again." When he took it the second time, he was looking for the change and noticed it at once.

St. John's wort can also improve the ability to stay alert, think clearly, concentrate, and cope with stress and other distractions. The following description given by a 43-year-old mother of two captures some of these effects. "It used to be, after 3 hours at work I was ready to take a nap," she said. "I couldn't concentrate on my tasks, and all the numbers that I was supposed to enter into reports seemed to blur together. But with St. John's wort, I don't get tired until about three in the afternoon, and then it's

Herb Quality Control

Even with reputable herb companies, it is still difficult to be sure that you are getting a quality product. The FDA closely scrutinizes drugs, but herbs are sold as food supplements and hence receive less careful scrutiny. Consumers may have good reason to wonder whether product labels match actual ingredients.

The supplement industry is averse to being regulated by the FDA because it believes the agency is biased in favor of pharmaceutical companies. However, the industry has not yet taken any serious steps to regulate itself in lieu of government regulation, which leaves consumers in a bind. Industrial Labs, a Denver-based company that is at the forefront of herb quality control, reported in 1997 that some of the raw St. John's wort available on a wholesale level wasn't St. John's wort at all, but an unknown plant spiked with synthetic hypericin.

---

no more than what anyone else feels. And when I get home, I still have energy to spare for my children."

A 30-year-old magazine editor put it this way: "I feel less scattered. It's like I have a better capacity to put my mind on task. Previously, I'd sink into a state of half-alert confusion, like my thinking was going one way and another at the same time. St. John's wort gives me enough extra mental energy to take charge of my own mind and make it do what I tell it."

St. John's wort can also improve energy levels indirectly. As an example, exercise is one of the best ways of increasing energy, but when you're depressed, you may find it difficult even to start. St. John's wort can help you

Not only is this fraudulent, it could also be dangerous. Hypericin probably isn't the active ingredient in St. John's wort, but it is the one that can cause sun sensitivity. (See chapter 7 for more details.) If very high levels of hypericin are added artificially, photosensitivity might become a real problem.

Some supplement manufacturers state that their products have been tested by independent laboratories. However, because it's the manufacturer who picks the laboratory, sends the samples, and reports the results, it isn't always clear whether such "independent" verification can be trusted completely. Nonetheless, until such time as a truly impartial body comes into being to evaluate the labeling accuracy of supplements, manufacturer-chosen laboratory analysis remains the best method of verification available.

to break this vicious cycle and improve your lifestyle, which will in turn provide additional benefits.

Besides enhanced energy, people who find St. John's wort helpful also typically report a lightening or elevation of mood. It isn't like a drug high, nor the almost mechanical happiness that some people say they experience on Prozac. Rather, it seems to more closely resemble the buoyancy of spirits that goes along with a normal good mood.

"I feel more playful now," one 27-year-old auto mechanic told me. "Instead of sinking down into a kind of drudgery, which is my normal state way too often, I want to have fun. At work I joke around with the other guys more, and at home I don't just sit around turning my problems over and over in my head. I get out and do stuff I like."

Another individual expressed his experience with St. John's wort this way: "It lifts my head out of the clouds. Although I don't usually get extremely depressed, I'm vaguely blue and down most of the time. I get by all right but I always seem to be unhappy about something. St. John's wort makes a big difference with that. Not that I don't ever get unhappy—I still do—but it isn't a constant thing. I go up and down more, instead of hugging the down side."

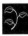

Due to the occasional side effect of stomach irritation, St. John's wort should be taken with food.

Another person described this effect as "increased emotional energy." He said that St. John's wort "not only makes my mind feel more alert, it helps me feel more strongly. Before I used to feel kind of numb and disconnected. On St. John's wort I get more excited, more involved with life."

Because the energizing and mood-elevating properties of St. John's wort occur without stimulant side effects, this treatment is often quite useful for depression accompanied by mild anxiety. As one person said, "Because I have more emotional energy, and I'm less gloomy, anxiety-provoking thoughts don't have as much power over me as they used to."

St. John's wort is not a tranquilizer; but by alleviating depression without producing artificial stimulation, it may produce a net effect of decreased anxiety. Some physicians recommend combining St. John's wort with mild herbal tranquilizers for additional benefit, as described in chapter 9.

Many people who take St. John's wort also report an improvement in sleep quality. Like the other effects of St. John's wort, this effect is gentle and "grows on you." After some period of taking the herb, many patients state that they sleep more soundly and restfully.

"My sleep seems deeper," a 23-year-old college student told me. "Before I used to hover near the surface most of the night, still processing my classes and turning my assignments over and over in my head. Now I feel like I go all the way under more of the time."

St. John's wort is typically standardized to 0.3% hypericin. A new type of product is standardized to 3 to 5% hyperforin.

However, St. John's wort does not directly induce sleep. The improvement in sleep quality appears to follow elimination of depression. In those cases when St. John's wort fails to alleviate depression (it certainly doesn't always succeed), sleep doesn't seem to improve either.

A similar connection also probably accounts for St. John's wort's positive influence on eating habits. People whose depression manifests as lack of desire for food frequently report improvement of appetite with the herb. This effect may be most notable in elderly people. One 70-year-old woman told me that when she started taking St. John's wort "food seemed to have more of a taste."

Depression can manifest as irritability rather than unhappiness. The daughter of the woman I just mentioned states unequivocally that "St. John's wort makes my mom a lot less grouchy. She doesn't get mad all the time."

Again, since St. John's wort is not a tranquilizer, this reduction of irritability is probably directly related to the alleviation of depression. The same effect is commonly seen with chemical antidepressants as well, although the side effects of drugs in the Prozac family can worsen appetite loss.

St. John's wort does not directly induce sleep, however, many patients who take St. John's wort report an improvement in sleep quality.

Self-esteem and ability to tolerate risk may also improve with St. John's wort. Taking the herb may also reduce shyness. The effect is seldom "miraculous," as is sometimes claimed for Prozac, but it's nonetheless detectable. Once more, St. John's wort's direct effect on depression seems to be at root.

As one man in his late 20s said, "Now that I have energy and feel fairly cheerful, I'm not so afraid to show my face in public. Before I didn't have much confidence that anyone would want to see me. I wouldn't have wanted to see me—I was always depressed. It's not like I've turned into Billy Crystal or anything now, but I feel like I have the inner *oomph* to get out there more."

The fact that St. John's wort is a natural herb plays a big role in some people's experience with it. For them, taking an herb *feels* much more acceptable than depending on a drug. "I hate being dependent on Prozac," is a comment I have heard dozens of times. "I feel like I'm some kind of sick person who needs medicine when I take drugs. It's an awful feeling," a 37-year-old carpenter said of her experience with Prozac. "But I don't mind taking St. John's wort. It's like taking a vitamin. It's a positive experience instead of an embarrassing one."

"Herbs are meant to be used for healing," another patient said. "Animals eat herbs when they don't feel well, too. It's a natural thing to take them, but Prozac isn't natural."

This attitude toward St. John's wort is based on feelings and intuitions, rather than cold facts. Those who do not share the underlying attitude often don't understand why herbs should be different from drugs. Doctors, for example, often tend to scoff at the notion of "natural." They point out that many drugs come from herbs, too.

While this is true, none of the chemical antidepressants come from herbs. They are all synthetic single chemicals. And St. John's wort, with its rich mixture of naturally occurring ingredients, simply feels more wholesome to people for whom that matters.

"I'm an environmentalist, too," said one of my patients. "I believe in sticking closer to nature whenever I can. I buy all cotton—I'd never dream of wearing polyester clothes. Taking an herb fits in with my lifestyle better."

The fact that St. John's wort is a natural herb plays a big role in some people's experience with it. For them, taking an herb feels much more acceptable than depending on a drug.

Just because something is natural, however, doesn't mean it's perfect. St. John's wort doesn't always succeed. Some people take it and feel no improvement at all. (The same thing happens with Prozac, of course, and more often than its reputation might suggest!) Others may think they feel an improvement and then decide after a while that it was wishful thinking.

For example, a 38-year-old physician colleague of mine tried St. John's wort and other alternative treatments for a full 2 years in what proved to be a vain attempt to treat his depression naturally. He frequently told me, "I think it's working now—I seem to be on an upswing," using the exact same words so often, it finally became a joke. When he finally tried Zoloft, the results were dramatic and indisputable. "I was just hoping it would work before," he said. "Zoloft is helping me in a way that I don't have to pinch myself to believe it."

Of course, Zoloft doesn't always work, either. It's not easy to come up with a figure on how often St. John's wort is beneficial for mild to moderate depression, but the research suggests a figure of 55%. As I've already said, this is a useful herb, not a miracle cure. It's a good tool for treating depression, and one that can satisfy the desire for "natural" treatment.

Don't Give Up Too Soon

You have to be patient when you take St. John's wort. The herb works gradually, typically taking 4 to 6 weeks to achieve its full effect. Dr. Rudolf Fritz Weiss, a physician sometimes called the father of German herbology, suggests giving the herb even more time to work. He says, "The mood lightening effect does not develop quickly—it is necessary to give the drug [St. John's wort] not just 4 weeks, but probably 2 or 3 months."[2] However, he goes on to say that "the first effects will usually be noted after 2 or 3 weeks."

Laura's story shows how easy it is to give up too early. She was a 43-year-old mother of three who had been plagued with depression her whole life. The cause was undoubtedly the shaming and verbal abuse that she experienced throughout her upbringing; but even after years of effective psychotherapy, her symptoms of depression lingered like a habit she couldn't break. Laura felt chronically blue, empty, and fatigued. Although she was never suicidal, she felt that she wasn't really living. The stresses of life left Laura so drained that by eight o'clock every night she didn't have enough energy left for anything but brushing her teeth and going to bed. Most weekends she spent lying on the couch whenever possible. "I'm coping and that's all I'm doing," she would say.

You have to be patient when you take St. John's wort. The herb works gradually, typically taking 4 to 6 weeks to achieve its full effect.

Laura's husband had been sympathetic, but he began spending more and more time apart from her. He wanted to take walks in the evening, play golf on the weekends, and go traveling from time to time. Although he would have preferred to do all these things with his wife, she was always too tired. He felt he needed to enjoy himself even if Laura couldn't join in. So he started to spend more time with his friends.

Laura felt that she and her husband were drifting apart. Her first response was to start going to sleep even earlier. Then something inside her woke up and told her she'd better do something positive before it was too late.

Laura's family doctor had been urging her for 2 years to try Prozac. Her particular kind of depression, with its chronic fatigue and excessive sleeping, seemed to make her a perfect candidate for this antidepressant. Laura had always demurred on the grounds that she didn't believe in taking drugs. However, now she felt ready to try anything. With a sigh of satisfaction, the doctor prescribed a single 20-mg dose of Prozac daily.

Unfortunately, things didn't go well. From the very first dose, Laura experienced unpleasant side effects. Her sleep, never restful, became broken and racked by nightmares. During the day she felt uneasy and on edge. She would startle violently when her husband entered the room unexpectedly or her 7-year-old screeched in play, and her heart would start racing and palpitating.

However, Laura did feel more energetic, and she began to get out with her husband more often. They took a trip to visit relatives in Minnesota, and once or twice they played golf on the weekends. For a little while she felt optimistic that their intimacy was returning, until the gradual development of sexual side effects rose up as a new obstacle. First orgasm became difficult, then impossible, and finally all desire disappeared. As Laura described the experience, "You'd think my body was made of wood the way it reacts. I don't feel anything. Sex is only a memory."

Sympathetic to her situation, Laura's doctor tried a succession of alternative medications. The results, unfortunately, were less than impressive. Paxil gave her headaches and made her more fatigued than ever, Zoloft caused exactly the same side effects as Prozac, Effexor made Laura "want to throw up night and day," and Serzone put her "into a trance so deep I didn't know if I was there or somewhere else."

And each time she stopped taking a drug, Laura sank back into her usual depression and the intolerable habits from constant fatigue. She felt trapped. She couldn't accept either her old depression or the side effects the drugs caused. It was in this state of frustration that she finally came to me.

"I don't know if there's anything that can help me without poisoning me," she said, "but if there is, I want to try it."

I started Laura on a standard dose of St. John's wort and asked her to come back once a week to tell me how she was doing. Strictly speaking, such frequent appointments aren't necessary, but I suspected she might give up on the herb without continual encouragement. I knew she was used to experiencing side effects, and I reasoned that she might misinterpret the gentleness of St. John's wort as ineffectiveness.

This fear proved justified when she came back for her first follow-up. "It's not doing anything," she said. "I'm back to my same old drudge of a self." When I asked her about side effects, she said, "Nothing, not a thing. I don't think there's anything in those capsules."

St. John's wort is not appropriate treatment for severe major depression.

I encouraged her to be patient. "You wanted a treatment that didn't cause side effects," I reminded her. "Now that you have it, don't give up before it has time to work. Remember, I said that you might have to wait 4 to 6 weeks."

My reassurance kept her going for another 2 weeks, but at the beginning of week 4, she was ready to throw in the towel. "I think I'm going to have to go back to drugs," she said.

It took all my powers of persuasion to keep her going. "I think I notice a difference in you already," I said, quite sincerely. "You don't look quite so depressed. I think you just can't recognize it because you're so used to feeling side effects along with feeling better."

It was something about her eyes that seemed different to me, but it wasn't until week 6 that Laura could notice the change herself. "It suddenly dawned on me the other day," she said, "that I don't feel so empty." I thought she looked considerably brighter and told her so.

By the eighth week it was obvious that St. John's wort was doing its job. "I feel like a human being when I get up in the morning," Laura said, smiling. "I have enough energy to enjoy myself. I'm not just getting by; I feel like I'm starting to live."

She was amazed at how gradually it all happened. "I couldn't tell anything at all for the longest time. But looking back I'd say that taking St. John's wort was like filling up a lake drop by drop. Almost without my being aware of it, the emptiness and hopelessness were gradually replaced by a quiet sense of calm."

On St. John's wort, Laura found a new ability to manage stress. "I can't believe how calm I feel. It's like I have a reservoir inside, something I can dip into when I need it. Before I was scraping the bottom of the barrel for something I didn't have."

How to Make the Change from Prescription Antidepressants

If you are taking medications for mild to moderate depression, you may be able to switch to St. John's wort if you prefer. Unfortunately, we don't know exactly how best to make this changeover.

The simplest way is to stop or taper off your medication, wait until it's out of your system, and then start the herb. With Prozac, up to 3 to 5 weeks may elapse before the drug is completely washed out. Other medications are fully excreted in a shorter time. Consult your doctor for information on how long you may need to wait.

The only problem with this method is that it may leave you feeling depressed for a little while. Many people overlap treatment for a week or two to try and avoid this problem, perhaps cutting their medication in half while starting St. John's wort. However, we don't know for sure whether it is safe to overlap medications and St. John's wort. No adverse effects have been officially reported, but there are reasons to believe there may be risks. The possible dangers of such combinations are described in the next chapter. I recommend consulting with your physician to obtain up-to-date information on this important subject.

Warning: If you are taking medications for severe depression, attempting a transition to St. John's wort is probably not appropriate.

When Not to Take St. John's Wort

St. John's wort is not appropriate treatment for severe, major depression. Most of the scientific studies of St. John's wort evaluated its effectiveness in mild to moderate depression (HAM-D scores of 24 or less). In the opinion of clinicians who use it, St. John's wort should not be relied upon for the treatment of severe depressive symptoms because its effects do not seem to be strong enough.

Major depression is a dangerous illness, and the risk of suicide is always present. In such cases medically supervised use of antidepressant drugs may be lifesaving (although this remains unproved).

Chapter 2 described the difference between severe and mild to moderate depression in detail. In general, the warning symptoms of severe, major depression include greatly decreased interest in normal activities, severe anxiety, severe insomnia, pronounced agitation or slowing down, overwhelming feelings of worthlessness, obsessive preoccupation with guilt, inability to cope with life, and most especially, significant suicidal thinking. St. John's wort is definitely not appropriate if you experience symptoms such as these. It's too gentle and gradual in its effects. I'd recommend taking medications, and soon.

St. John's wort may also not be appropriate treatment between major depressions for people who suffer from

Lucy's Story

L ucy's story is a good example of when not to take St. John's wort.

This 33-year-old retail clerk came to my office requesting St. John's wort, but she went out with a prescription for Prozac and a referral to a psychiatrist. She was tearful from the moment she walked in, and her story further showed me the depths of her depression.

"I try to think positive," she said, "but I feel so hopeless and worthless. I've even thought of taking my husband's hunting rifle and shooting myself." After she said this, she burst into tears.

It didn't take me more than about 5 seconds to recognize that St. John's wort was not for Lucy. Constant crying, overwhelming feelings of worthlessness and guilt, and, most especially, frequent and realistic thoughts of suicide mean that depression has gone too far for St. John's wort.

frequent major depressive episodes. While research indicates that continuous antidepressant drug treatment can prevent recurrence, St. John's wort is probably not powerful enough to provide the equivalent benefit.

The only time St. John's wort should be used in severe depression is when all other antidepressants have failed. Occasionally, but just occasionally, it may work.

An important final point is that symptoms resembling depression can be caused by a wide variety of medical illnesses, including thyroid conditions, anemia, and asthma. It is important to exclude such physical causes of depression before turning to self-treatment with St. John's wort.

I explained to Lucy that she had fallen too deeply into depression to benefit from herbal medicine. "St. John's wort isn't strong enough," I said. "You need something like Prozac, and I want you to see a psychiatrist this afternoon. I'm afraid you're going to hurt yourself otherwise."

Like many others in the depths of major depression, Lucy found dramatic relief through antidepressant drugs, and the medication may have saved her life. Fifteen percent of people who suffer from major depression commit suicide. Although it's difficult to find hard evidence to show that antidepressants actually reduce the incidence of suicide, it certainly seems that they do. Drug treatment usually produces a dramatic turn-around in severe major depression, and suicidal thoughts are often one of the first symptoms to improve. St. John's wort is not a good treatment when depression is this severe.

Don't Forget to Treat the Whole Person

We are a pill-happy society, and to substitute St. John's wort as a natural pill instead of a chemical one is to miss a large part of the picture. Illustrating this point very well in *Listening to Prozac,* Peter Kramer states, "The patients I medicate with Prozac tend first to have undergone extensive courses of psychotherapy. . . . There needs to be a readiness for Prozac, [which] works best in patients whose conflicts are resolved but whose biologically autonomous handicaps remain."

In other words, if a person has done his or her psychological work, but remains held back by moods that seem connected to built-in brain chemistry, the use of a drug (or herb) may be helpful. But pills shouldn't be used as the sole and single remedy for depression.

Besides diet, other lifestyle issues can make a significant impact on depression. Exercise, enjoyable activities, a comfortable living situation, satisfactory employment, tolerable levels of stress, and good relationships with friends and family are all important.

Many of us suffer from complex and stubborn emotional binds that cannot be simply alleviated by taking a substance. Rather, it is often necessary to tease apart these constrictions, to loosen their grip, and to soften their imperious domination. It takes a skillful and sensitive psychotherapist to accomplish this, not a tablet.

Yet, for some people, even years of excellent psychotherapy fail to relieve depression. They seem prey to moods that have a life of their own, as much physically built-in as brown hair or blue eyes.

We don't really know for sure whether mild to moderate depression is genetically inheritable. It may be that depressive habits of mind are passed along just like mannerisms or figures of speech. If all members of a family tend to say "please" when they don't understand something they've heard (like everyone on my wife's side), we don't attribute this shared habit to DNA. We understand that they all simply learned the habit together.

Similarly, depression may be to some extent learned by imitation. Children may notice parental patterns of unhappiness and adopt them for their own. But in some people it appears that genetics must play a role. No matter how hard they try to compensate or cope, no matter how many bad emotional habits they solve through psychotherapy, depressive moods prevail. These are the people who find antidepressant therapy most helpful, and St. John's wort may be helpful for them, too. Still, such treatments work best after the hard work of psychotherapy has been completed.

Besides psychotherapy, there are many other commonsense approaches to treating depression that shouldn't be neglected in favor of antidepressants. I already mentioned the necessity of excluding physical diseases that may masquerade as depression, such as low thyroid. It is also important to consider basic lifestyle issues.

Poor diet can certainly increase symptoms of depression. There is a strong clinical impression, and at least some double-blind evidence, that in some people, caffeine and sugar can produce symptoms of depression.[3] Numerous vitamin and mineral deficiencies can cause depression, as well. Low levels of folic acid, vitamin B_{12}, pyridoxine, iron, and magnesium are some of the most commonly implicated nutritional influences on depression.

Besides diet, other lifestyle issues can make a significant impact on depression. Exercise, enjoyable activities, a comfortable living situation, satisfactory employment, tolerable levels of stress, and good relationships with friends and family are all important.

I remember one 30-year-old woman who had tried both antidepressants and St. John's wort without success. Her depression lifted only after she left her mother's home and moved into her own house. Interestingly, this solution was suggested, not by her therapist or myself, but by her 7-year-old niece!

People sometimes tell me that they have tried commonsense changes and received no benefit, so they went back to their former unhealthy lifestyle. I often suggest revisiting the issue. With the additional help offered through the use of St. John's wort, solutions that were previously attempted without results may become more effective. The same may be true of psychotherapy: The mood and energy boost of an antidepressant, whether natural or otherwise, may facilitate progress.

The best approach to treating depression (and addressing any other problem) is to look at the whole picture. Taking into account medical, psychological, and lifestyle issues, St. John's wort may make an important contribution to a comprehensive solution.

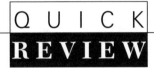

- The proper dose of St. John's wort is 300 mg 3 times daily (or 600 mg in the morning and 300 mg in the evening) of a dose standardized to contain 0.3% hypericin. New products may be standardized to 3 to 5% hyperiform.

- To avoid the occasional side effect of stomach irritation, take St. John's wort with meals. I recommend purchasing either a product certified in Germany or one made in the United States according to European manufacturing standards.

- Results generally take several weeks to develop. Remember that St. John's wort is only effective for mild to moderate depression, and will not work for severe major depression.

- If you are taking antidepressant drugs and wish to switch to St. John's wort, you should seek a physician's supervision.

Safety Issues

Among patients who visit family practitioners' offices, depression is far more common than high blood pressure, according to at least one study.[1] Depression is a prevalent and largely under-treated illness. Every year, at least 15 million Americans experience major depression, and the number who experience chronic depressive symptoms of a mild to moderate nature is undoubtedly even higher. Depression costs society tens of billions of dollars. In addition to their direct health-care costs, people who are depressed miss more work than the rest of the population and experience five times the rate of disability.[2]

More important than any dollar figure, however, is the fact that depression causes a tremendous amount of human suffering. According to one study, the loss of well-being and physical capacity caused by depression typically exceeds the negative effects of diabetes, back pain, and arthritis.[3] It decreases the ability to enjoy life, impairs child-rearing, cramps social relationships, interferes with healthy lifestyle habits, and inhibits career success. Furthermore, depression's vague symptoms frequently cause extended and aggressive medical examinations and testing.

There is no question that Prozac and other antidepressant drugs have improved the lives of many depressed people. But the fear of these drugs' side effects has kept many people from seeking treatment. It is precisely here that St. John's wort shows its greatest value.

St. John's Wort's Excellent Side-Effect Profile

St. John's wort is nearly side-effect–free. Overall, a total of 4,450 people taking St. John's wort have been screened for side effects. This closely matches the 4,000 individuals who received Prozac in premarketing studies (according to the 1997 *PDR*).[4]

In one study of 3,250 patients taking St. John's wort extract for 4 weeks, the most common side effect was mild stomach discomfort, and it occurred in only 0.6% of patients taking the herb.[5] Allergic reactions such as skin rash and itching developed in 0.5%, tiredness in 0.4%, and restlessness in 0.3%. Other side effects occurred at still lower rates. Only 1.5% of the participants dropped out of the study due to perceived side effects, and the total percentage of participants reporting side effects was 2.4.

Among the approximately 1,200 individuals observed in St. John's wort versus placebo trials, the overall incidence of side effects was 4.1%.[6] (A 19.8% side-effect rate is mentioned in the abstract of the *British Medical Journal* overview.[7] However, this is an artificially inflated number, as explained in the next chapter.)

Toxicity

St. John's wort is a very safe herb. In the extensive German experience with St. John's wort as a treatment for depression, there have been no published reports of serious adverse consequences.[8]

One way to judge the ultimate safety of a substance is to give progressively higher doses to animals and see how high you have to go to kill half of them. This dose is then reported as the LD50, or lethal dose in 50%. To adjust for the size of the animal, this dose is usually stated in proportion to body weight. For Prozac, the dose is 248 mg/kg in mice and 452 mg/kg in rats. This is a pretty high dose as far as drugs go, making Prozac one of the safer medications in wide use.

However, researchers haven't even been able to identify a lethal dose of St. John's wort. In studies of mice, rats, and dogs treated for 26 weeks, 50% fatalities were not observed even at dosages as enormous as 5,000 mg/kg.[9] There was no evidence of carcinogenic activity either. Considering that people ordinarily take about 15 mg/kg daily, it is clear that St. John's wort has a very high margin of safety.

Theoretical Warnings

Numerous books and articles on St. John's wort mention two serious problems as real possibilities: photosensitivity and MAO inhibitor–like reactions to foods. These theoretical risks are essentially never observed in practice; but because they are so widely discussed and have frightened some people away from using St. John's wort, I shall explore them here.

Photosensitivity?

Certain drugs significantly increase the risk of sunburn. Individuals taking sulfa antibiotics, tetracycline, various diuretics, and even tricyclic antidepressants can sometimes develop severe blistering sunburn after relatively short exposure. This potentially deadly phenomenon is called *photosensitivity* or, when severe, *phototoxicity.* People tak-

...osensitizing drugs are supposed to stay indoors or, if they must go out, use effective sunblock.

There are some similar concerns about St. John's wort. Back in the eighteenth century, light-skinned cattle and sheep grazing on large quantities of St. John's wort were observed to develop severe, blistering sunburns. Ranchers in Oregon and Washington apparently lost millions of dollars' worth of livestock due to sunburn during the "Klamath weed" infestation of St. John's wort in the Pacific Northwest (as described in chapter 1).

The sun-sensitizing toxin in St. John's wort is the same hypericin listed on standardized extracts of the herb. However, the quantity of hypericin required to cause photosensitivity is believed to be significantly more than the recommended dosage.[10]

Photosensitivity has not occurred in a single person involved in studies investigating St. John's wort as a treatment for depression, nor have any published reports of photosensitivity emerged out of the widespread use of this herb in Germany. However, in a recent study, sun-sensitive people who were given twice the normal dose of St. John's wort did sunburn a little bit faster when they were treated with artificial UV radiation.[11] Individuals given

Photosensitivity has not occurred in a single person involved in studies investigating St. John's wort as a treatment for depression, nor have any published reports of photosensitivity emerged out of the widespread use of this herb in Germany.

high-dose intravenous synthetic hypericin in AIDS experiments have also shown photosensitivity.

It is always possible that a few people might sunburn faster on normal oral doses of St. John's wort too. Therefore, extremely sun-sensitive people should perhaps use extra caution when they start taking this herb, exposing themselves to sun (and artificial UV) cautiously at first. High-altitude sun exposure may be the most likely type of exposure to cause a problem.

MAO Inhibitor–Related Side Effects?

The official German monograph on St. John's wort suggests that individuals taking the herb should observe precautions similar to those necessary with MAO inhibitors. However, this is a theoretical warning. There isn't a single published case report of MAO inhibitor–type reactions occurring in people taking St. John's wort for depression.

As you may recall from the previous chapter, people on MAO inhibitors must be very careful about what they eat. Cheese, wine, yeast, and other tyramine-containing foods can cause serious, even fatal, reactions. A variety of drugs can trigger the same reaction, including Sudafed (pseudoephedrine), phenylpropanolamine, and other nasal decongestants.

This potential interaction makes MAO inhibitors rather dangerous drugs. The same warning has been associated with St. John's wort, not because such an interaction has ever been observed, but because of one study performed in 1984 that suggested St. John's wort could inhibit monoamine-oxidase.

Subsequent studies failed to substantiate these MAO inhibitor–like effects. As explained earlier, the MAO theory of St. John's wort has fallen into disfavor, to be replaced by a serotonin-based hypothesis. Thus the only basis for fearing MAO inhibitor–type reactions has been

..ly refuted. The 1996 *British Medical Journal* re-
v.. St. John's wort[12] did not even mention MAO inhibition. This is simply not a real risk.

Drug Interactions

Individuals considering taking an herb for any purpose commonly ask whether it could interfere with medication they are taking. Because drugs frequently interfere with one another, this is a realistic and sensible concern. Unfortunately, the question is difficult to answer with any certainty.

There are no known interactions between St. John's wort and pharmaceutical medications. However, this statement should not be taken to imply that no such interactions exist. It is certainly possible that unrecognized problems may occur in certain people, because systematic trials have never been performed to look for drug-herb interactions.

Much the same situation exists in the world of drugs. Medical researchers do not go down the list of available drugs and try them in every possible combination. It would be too expensive and time-consuming, and deliberately exposing people in clinical trials to unnecessary medications would be unethical, as well. Drug interactions are usually discovered by accident or by analogy with already discovered drug interactions.

What can be said for certain is this: In the extensive German experience with St. John's wort, no reports of problems caused by the simultaneous use of St. John's wort and a pharmaceutical drug have ever been published.[13]

Some authorities have warned that combining St. John's wort with serotonin-raising drugs such as Prozac might cause a dangerous rise in serotonin levels, producing what is called "serotonergic syndrome." However, once again this is a theoretical warning, based on the unproven supposition that St. John's wort works like Prozac by increasing serotonin. Such a problem has never been officially reported. However, to be on the safe side, I recommend consulting with a physician before overlapping St. John's wort with standard antidepressants. Note also that some antidepressants stay in the blood for quite a long time after you stop them, most especially Prozac (3 to 5 weeks). If you make the switch from Prozac to St. John's wort, before starting the St. John's wort, you will have to give yourself several weeks of no treatment at all to avoid combined treatment.

There has also recently been a report that St. John's wort may lower blood levels of theophylline, an asthma medication. Unpublished data from the University of Colorado suggests that the hypericin in St. John's wort may increase the activity of an enzyme called cytochrome P-450.[14,15]

This substance is responsible for metabolizing many drugs and other chemicals. By increasing P-450 activity, St. John's wort may cause the body

Preliminary studies suggest that St. John's wort may interfere with drugs that are affected by cytochrome P-450 CYP 1A1 and 1A2 induction, as well as certain cancer chemotherapy drugs. Ask your physician for more information.

to break down these drugs faster, thereby decreasing their effectiveness. Before taking St. John's wort, it might be a good idea to ask your doctor if any of your medications would be affected by "cytochrome P-450 CYP 1A1 and 1A2 induction."

Long-Term Safety

A question people commonly ask about St. John's wort is whether it is safe to take for many years in a row. This is a legitimate concern because many drugs cause problems that only become evident after a long period of use, and herbs could conceivably do the same thing.

Unfortunately, there has never been a study formally evaluating the safety of St. John's wort over a period exceeding 8 weeks. Wide usage in Germany over the last 10 years has failed to reveal any delayed harmful effects, but this does not mean that there couldn't be hidden, subtle, or occasional side effects that simply haven't yet been noticed. Thus it is impossible to make a definitive statement that St. John's wort is safe over the long term.

The same lack of knowledge prevails for Prozac, other antidepressants, and indeed virtually all medical therapies. The only absolutely foolproof way to determine whether or not long-

Another study out of the University of Colorado suggests that St. John's wort may interfere with the action of the antitumor drugs etoposide (VePesid), teniposide (Vumon), mitoxantrone (Novantrone), and doxorubicin (Adriamycin).[16]

Is St. John's Wort Safe During Pregnancy and While Nursing?

Like answering the question of long-term risks, establishing safety during pregnancy and while nursing is very difficult. Drug companies are reluctant to state that any drug can be used safely during pregnancy and nursing because

term harm exists would be to take two identical populations, give one half the drug and the other half placebo, and keep the experiment going for decades. If after 50 years or so no problems cropped up in the treated group, one could then conclude that a treatment was absolutely safe in the long run.

Obviously, such an experiment has never been done, whether for drugs, herbs, vaccinations, food preservatives, or foods. Thus the long-term safety of all treatments must be regarded as not established.

Some people feel that because St. John's wort is a natural herb it is more likely to be safe in the long run than a drug, but this is an emotional statement rather than a rational one. Numerous herbs have been shown to be potentially toxic, including comfrey and chaparral. For that matter, barbecued hamburger appears to be carcinogenic. In other words, there is no guarantee that St. John's wort is safe just because it's natural.

there is no way to be sure without trying it, and that may run unacceptable risks. The same may be said for St. John's wort. Although there is no evidence that this herb should be avoided during pregnancy and nursing, no absolute statement as to its safety can be made, either.

Is St. John's Wort Safe for Children?

This is another question that can't be answered with certainty. All the studies of St. John's wort were performed with adult participants, so all one can really say is that its safety for children is not known.

Is St. John's Wort Safe for Those with Liver or Kidney Disease?

Because the body processes most substances through the liver or kidneys, people with diseases in these organs frequently must exercise special cautions in the use of drugs. Whether similar precautions should apply to St. John's wort has not been discovered.

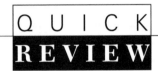

- St. John's wort appears to be nearly side-effect–free. Occasionally, it produces mild stomach upset or allergic reactions (mainly skin rash). Enormous doses have been given to animals without harmful effects.

- Contrary to early reports, St. John's wort is not believed to be an MAO inhibitor, and the usual MAO-inhibitor warnings (avoid cheese, decongestants, etc.) do not apply. Overdoses of St. John's wort may cause increased sensitivity to the sun.

- For theoretical reasons, it may not be safe to combine St. John's wort with other antidepressant medications. Since Prozac stays in the system for several weeks after it is discontinued, you may need to let it wash out of your system for a month or more before starting St. John's wort.

- Preliminary studies suggest that St. John's wort may interfere with drugs that are affected by cytochrome P-450 CYP 1A1 and 1A2 induction, as well as with certain cancer chemotherapy drugs. Ask your physician for more information.

- The safety of St. John's wort in children, pregnant or nursing mothers, or those with liver or kidney disease has not been established.

How St. John's Wort Compares with Conventional Medications

T he preceding chapters detailed the scientific evidence suggesting that St. John's wort is an effective treatment for mild to moderate depression and (at recommended doses) is also relatively side-effect–free. The studies from which this conclusion is drawn are scientifically sound, involve reasonably high numbers of participants, and are published in reputable European journals.

However, none of the studies quoted thus far directly compared the effectiveness of St. John's wort against pharmaceutical options. This chapter explores the question: Which is the more appropriate treatment for mild to moderate depression, St. John's wort or antidepressant drugs? (See table 1 and table 2 for summaries of relevant information regarding St. John's wort and conventional medications.) Unfortunately, as we shall see, there is not enough data to draw a firm conclusion.

Table 1. St. John's Wort

Presumed Action	Benefits	Possible Side Effects
inhibits serotonin, norepinephrine, and dopamine reuptake	helpful for mild to moderate depression minimal side effects	digestive distress (rare) allergic reactions (rare) photosensitivity (in overdose only)

Direct Comparisons

In 1993 E. Vorbach and colleagues performed an experiment designed to compare the effectiveness of St. John's wort and imipramine in the treatment of mild to moderate depression.[1] Imipramine is the oldest of the tricyclic drugs, and it is used relatively seldom in present clinical practice because of its many side effects. Its efficacy has never been surpassed, however, and imipramine remains the "gold standard" against which newer antidepressants are usually compared.

When Eli Lilly was trying to get Prozac approved, the company sponsored extensive clinical comparisons between its new medication and imipramine. The results did not show that Prozac was more powerful than imipramine. Rather, all they demonstrated was comparable effectiveness, which was sufficient for the FDA.

Vorbach chose to compare St. John's wort against the same gold standard. He and his fellow researchers prepared tablets of St. John's wort extract that were identical to imipramine in appearance, flavor, and consistency. Participants were then randomized into two groups, one receiving 300 mg of standardized St. John's wort 3 times daily and the other receiving 25 mg of imipramine 3 times daily. A total of 135 patients at 20 separate physicians' practices were enrolled in the study and followed for 6 weeks. The age range was 18 to 75 years, and male and female patients were included in about equal proportion.

Using the HAM-D index, physicians rated participants' levels of depression at the beginning of the study and at 2-week intervals until the end. Individuals' levels of depression were also monitored with a separate scale known as the Clinical Global Impressions scale (CGI). This scale allows a somewhat different perspective on the progress of depression. The recorded progression of these scores provides a direct comparison between the antidepressant powers of imipramine and those of St. John's wort.

For both mild and moderate depression, St. John's wort seems at least roughly comparable to drug treatment.

At the beginning of the study, HAM-D scores for both groups of individuals averaged about 20. Those treated with St. John's wort improved their scores by 55%, while those taking imipramine only improved by 45%. At the end of the test, 81.8% of the participants on St. John's wort were rated as "significantly improved" according to the CGI, while only 62.5% of those on imipramine received that score.

Because the differences between these numbers were not large enough to be statistically significant, the study's conclusion was this: St. John's wort and imipramine are equally effective in the treatment of mild to moderate depression. Since imipramine is known to be as effective as Prozac, it seems logical to assume that St. John's wort would also prove as effective as Prozac if they were matched head-to-head.

Table 2. Comparison of Conventional
Drug Antidepressants

Presumed Action	Benefits	Possible Side Effects
Prozac		
inhibits serotonin reuptake	low toxicity; effective for major depression;useful in mild to moderate depression usually non-sedating few or no side effects in many cases	nausea loss of appetite anorgasmia in women impotence in men decreased libido insomnia nervousness tremors tiredness asthenia dry mouth sweating
Zoloft		
similar to Prozac	often not as stimulating as Prozac, otherwise similar to Prozac (between Prozac and Paxil)	same as Prozac
Paxil		
similar to Prozac	less stimulating than Prozac on average, otherwise, same as Prozac	same as Prozac fatigue

Table 2. Comparison of Conventional Drug Antidepressants *(continued)*

Presumed Action	Benefits	Possible Side Effects
Luvox		
similar to Prozac	less stimulating than Prozac on average, otherwise, same as Prozac	same as Prozac fatigue
Effexor		
inhibits serotonin and norepinephrine reuptake	effective for major depression. May be useful for mild to moderate depression	similar to Prozac, Paxil, and Luvox nausea apparently less impairment of sexual function than Prozac
Trazodone		
inhibits serotonin reuptake	helpful for insomnia Other Comments: Generally too sedating to be useful in mild to moderate depression	severe drowsiness dizziness fatigue nervousness dry mouth headache possible severe priapism

(continues)

Table 2. Comparison of Conventional Drug Antidepressants *(continued)*

Presumed Action	Benefits	Possible Side Effects
Serzone		
inhibits reuptake of serotonin and norepinephrine	does not interfere with sexual function. May be useful for anxiety Other Comments: Generally too sedating to be useful in mild to moderate depression	headache sleepiness dizziness asthenia dry mouth nausea constipation
Wellbutrin		
weakly inhibits reuptake of serotonin, norepinephrine, and dopamine	does not interfere with sexual function. Effective in major depression. May be useful in mild to moderate depression	nausea dry mouth dizziness insomnia agitation restlessness anxiety seizures at high doses

Table 2. Comparison of Conventional Drug Antidepressants

Presumed Action	Benefits	Possible Side Effects

Tricyclics (Tofranil, Pamelor, Elavil, Sinequan, Ludiomil)

Presumed Action	Benefits	Possible Side Effects
inhibits reuptake of serotonin and norepinephrine	effective for major depression works rapidly (Maprotiline only) Other Comments: Generally too sedating to be useful in mild to moderate depression	fatigue drowsiness dry mouth dizziness blurred vision sexual dysfunction constipation sweating heart palpitations weight gain urinary retention cardiac injury at high doses

MAO inhibitors (Marplan, Naril, Parnate)

Presumed Action	Benefits	Possible Side Effects
poisons monoamineoxidase, inhibits breakdown of amines	sometimes successful when other drugs fail Other Comments: Too risky for use in mild to moderate depression	insomnia dizziness sexual dysfunction dangerous with certain foods and over-the-counter drugs

Unfortunately, there is a serious flaw in this otherwise excellent piece of research: The dosage of imipramine was too low. Participants received 75 mg of imipramine daily and no more, while in real clinical practice, doses of 150 to 250 mg are frequently necessary to achieve optimum results. One study that compared imipramine to Zoloft settled on an average dose of about 200 mg of imipramine per day.[2] In other words, the 75 mg used for this St. John's wort comparison study may simply have been too low to display imipramine's full powers.

For American physicians, a study where participants were given only 75 mg of imipramine simply doesn't prove very much. It almost seems to show that St. John's wort isn't very effective after all, if it only matches such a low dose of the drug. From the point of view of validating the comparative power of St. John's wort, this study is a disaster.

However, the researchers who performed this study were not fools. Vorbach knew he was using a low dose of imipramine, and did so for a very interesting reason. He wanted to keep the double-blind structure of the study intact.

Imipramine causes a number of significant and obvious side effects, such as dry mouth, dizziness, and sedation, and the higher the dose the stronger the side effects. In comparison, St. John's wort produces next to none. If Vorbach had used imipramine in full doses, participants receiving the drug instead of the herb would almost undoubtedly have been able to guess which group they were in. The examining physicians would also have been able to figure it out, and the whole purpose of the double-blind setup would have been negated. As described in chapter 4, when the blind is broken by side-effects, the potential influence of placebo creeps in and the study isn't fully valid. This is a consideration often ignored by U.S. researchers. I hope that the NIH scientists comparing Zoloft to St. John's wort take this problem into account.

Vorbach felt that his results should be meaningful despite the low dose of imipramine. In Germany, many physicians believe that even 50 mg of imipramine should be adequate for most outpatients. However, most physicians in the United States would not agree.

A similar trial (with a similar flaw) was performed by G. Harrer and colleagues in 1993.[3] It compared the effectiveness of St. John's wort against that of another tricyclic antidepressant: maprotiline. Maprotiline is an interesting antidepressant for two reasons. Unlike most tricyclics, it is a highly specific drug. It elevates levels of norepinephrine but does not change serotonin at all. This makes it the opposite of Prozac, which raises serotonin without affecting norepinephrine. Maprotiline is also unusual in its exceptionally rapid onset of action. Most people who take it experience a reduction in symptoms of depression after only 1 or 2 weeks, compared to the typical 4 to 6 weeks most other antidepressants require.

Harrer's study enrolled 102 participants at 6 doctors' practices and followed them for 4 weeks. The participants were both male and female and ranged in age from 24 to 65 years old. On average, their initial HAM-D scores were about 21, representing moderate depression.

Half the individuals were given St. John's wort and the other half maprotiline. The HAM-D rating was then repeated at the end of week 2 and week 4. As expected, maprotiline was the early leader, producing more marked improvements at the first retest. However, by 4 weeks St. John's wort had fully caught up with maprotiline's benefit. In both groups, the final improvement in HAM-D scores was essentially the same: about 50%.

Nonetheless, there was one significant difference between those given St. John's wort and those treated with maprotiline. According to the CGI, a higher percentage of individuals taking the herb were evaluated as "very much improved" or "no longer ill" compared to those taking the drug. The researchers felt that this difference was probably due to the side effects caused by maprotiline.

Once again, while the results were impressive, their validity is undercut by the low drug dosage used in the study. Participants received only 75 mg of maprotiline a day. In normal clinical practice, this is only a starting dose for the drug. Physicians usually push the level upward to achieve optimum effects. A typical final dose might be 100 to 150 mg daily.

In almost all studies of St. John's wort, the incidence of side effects is extremely low.

In reviewing all the St. John's wort versus tricyclic drug studies, an editorial in the *British Medical Journal* expressed a wish that "the comparator should be tested in therapeutic doses" and refused to take the results seriously.[4]

One recent study did use doses of imipramine high enough to treat mild to moderate depression (150 mg daily).[5] However, this study enrolled individuals with severe depression (HAM-D scores above 25). In such cases, a dose of imipramine as high as 250 to 300 mg would be commonly used. A total of 209 individuals were followed for 6 weeks in a randomized, double-blind multicenter trial. St. John's wort was given at double doses, but still did not perform quite as well as imipramine. Thus, this study appears to indicate that St. John's wort is not as effective as standard antidepressants in the treatment of severe major depression. This should come as no surprise, as St. John's wort has never been seriously suggested as a treatment for severe depression.

Indirect Comparisons

There is another way to evaluate the relative effectiveness of St. John's wort and drug therapy: Compare the drop in

HAM-D scores that each treatment produces in its own separate trials. Such a method resembles comparing runners' times when racing alone. Direct head-to-head competition defines the winner more conclusively, but individual records can be used to qualify potential competitors for the real match. Similarly, while not scientifically rigorous, cross-study comparisons can give us a clue as to whether St. John's wort is a realistic contender.

To ensure this comparison is between apples and apples, not apples and oranges, all studies described following used the same 17-item HAM-D test in their evaluations of results. I focus here on trials involving the newer antidepressant drugs because those are the ones most frequently prescribed for individuals with mild to moderate depression.

One Prozac study evaluated 372 participants with mild depression (HAM-D scores of 15 to 19), but the results were not very impressive.[6] Placebo-treated and Prozac-treated participants experienced essentially identical improvements in HAM-D scores. In other words, Prozac proved on average to be no more effective than a sugar pill for treating mild depression.

Faced with these negative results, the authors of the study resorted to questionable statistical manipulations. They looked closely at the responses of each individual and identified a subgroup that responded well to Prozac. Their conclusion was that Prozac is definitely effective for certain people with mild depression and not others.

Actually, this form of statistical reasoning is highly dubious. If two contestants are pitching pennies and come to a draw, it's always possible to pick out a few selected tosses and say, "Contestant two was much better with certain pennies than contestant one." Such a statement really communicates nothing except to reiterate the normal action of the laws of chance. A draw is a draw, even if there are a few brilliant tosses along the way.

Thus Prozac's mediocre results in this study suggest that it is not a terribly effective treatment for mild depression. A comparable study of St. John's wort in treating mild depression showed better results.[7] In this trial of 105 patients with HAM-D scores averaging about 16, participants were given either St. John's wort or placebo. Those receiving St. John's wort demonstrated an average improvement rate almost twice as high as for those taking placebo.

This evidence appears to suggest that St. John's wort is effective for a broader spectrum of mildly depressed individuals than Prozac is. However, this comparison cannot be taken as scientifically solid, because the individuals in the St. John's wort group were not identical to those in the Prozac study. One difference was that the St. John's wort participants were chosen on the basis of older, looser definitions of depression than the relatively rigorous *DSM* criteria that the Prozac researchers used. Also, the first trial was conducted in the United States, the other in Germany. Numerous cultural and demographic differences may thus confound the results.

Another relevant study followed a total of 416 outpatients with average HAM-D scores of about 13.[8] Participants were randomly assigned to receive either Zoloft, imipramine, or placebo. Both the Zoloft- and imipramine-treated groups showed a statistically significant response to treatment, and the results were quite similar to what was achieved by St. John's wort in the study just described.

However, once again, differences in participant population weaken the power of this comparison study, as well. The situation is analogous to runners from different countries establishing records in their own homeland, under different conditions of weather, altitude, and terrain. Numerous subtle factors make a precise comparison of speed impossible. Nonetheless, what *can* be said for certain regarding treatment of mild depression is that St. John's wort is definitely a contender.

This discussion involved individuals with mild depression. It is more difficult to find drug studies to compare against St. John's wort studies for those with *moderate* depression. There is plenty of research into St. John's wort for moderately depressed people. However, the Eli Lilly company was unable to provide me with any studies that evaluated Prozac in a similar population. The best I could do was to find a study that evaluated people with moderate depression when they were given either placebo or the tricyclic drug desipramine.[9] The results showed a success rate of 55%.

This figure is exactly the same as the overall effectiveness of St. John's wort when results of all studies of the herb are combined.[10] Thus, for both mild and moderate depression, St. John's wort seems at least roughly comparable to drug treatment.

People given placebo typically develop side effects at remarkable levels when they think they may be taking a real drug. Thus, the high rate of side effects seen in St. John's wort versus drug tests are probably falsely inflated.

What Doctors Say

The research just described, while suggestive, is far from definitive. To flesh out a picture of the relative power of St. John's wort and drugs, let's now turn to the clinical impression of physicians familiar with the herb.

Let's Be Fair, Part I

Alternative medicine is frequently (and often fairly) criticized for being less scientific than conventional medicine. However, sometimes the reverse is true. A good example is the criticism often leveled against St. John's wort that it hasn't been properly studied as a treatment for severe depression. But the fact is, no one is recommending it for severe depression. All its advocates recommend the herb only for mild to moderate depression.

On the other hand, Prozac is widely prescribed for mild to moderate depression. However, an examination of the research record shows that it hasn't been properly studied for mild to moderate depression. So actually it's Prozac that's being used unscientifically in this case.

The influential German physician Dr. Rudolf Weiss says, "The antidepressant effect [of St. John's wort] is not so unequivocal and intensive as those of modern synthetic antidepressants."[11]

This view is shared by other clinicians who use St. John's wort. Dr. John Motl, a psychiatrist with extensive experience in alternative treatments, told me that St. John's wort is milder in its effects than Prozac. "I wouldn't use it for major depression," he said. "But in mild to moderate depression it can be very helpful."

Based on my own experience, I would agree. I have seen several people attempt to self-treat severe depression with St. John's wort, but none were successful. In each case chemical antidepressants proved significantly more effective.

Even though St. John's wort is weaker than drug treatment for serious depression, this doesn't mean that it is comparatively less effective in mild to moderate depression. The studies described in the previous section seem to suggest that the benefits are roughly equal.

Nonetheless, many physicians believe that even in mild to moderate depression, drugs are more powerful than St. John's wort. This is the impression of Scott Shannon, the Colorado psychiatrist I mentioned earlier. "Drugs are usually stronger," he says, "but I frequently try St. John's wort first because of the better side-effect profile."

My own experience suggests that Prozac and similar drugs are a bit more potent than St. John's wort for mild to moderate depression. Those who try antidepressant medications seem to report dramatic results more often than those who use the herb. However, I'm not sure I trust my own impression. We may all be under the influence of the power of suggestion.

My own evaluations may have been subconsciously affected by the media hype over Prozac. Do I—and Scott Shannon and others in the medical field—unconsciously expect superior results from drug treatment and thereby convey more confidence to our patients when we prescribe medications? Does this same bias also skew our informal evaluation of patient improvement? I'm not sure.

Mild to moderate depression is such a fluid and subjective illness that it leaves plenty of room for the power of suggestion to act on both doctors and patients. The entire situation is murky. Some people may respond to the fame of Prozac and experience especially positive results because they expect to experience them. The effect can go the other way, too, however. Some of my patients distrust drugs on general principle and are loath to accept that they might ever receive benefit from one. Since they are far more comfortable with natural herbs, this emotional bias might very well affect their response to treatment.

Perhaps this is why St. John's wort is the antidepressant of choice in Germany. There, both physicians' and patients' attitudes are strongly sympathetic to the use of herbal medications and less impressed by the power of drugs. St. John's wort may benefit from a topspin of positive feeling in Germany, just as Prozac does on this side of the ocean.

St. John's wort gives a wholesome message. Psychologically speaking, it "feels" more like a food than a drug; it is a natural plant rather than a synthetic chemical.

The double-blind study was developed by medical researchers in order to eliminate the effects of suggestion. If the true identity of treatment or placebo is concealed from both physicians and participants, the results should be more reliable. When it comes to antidepressant drugs, however, the usual precautions may not be sufficient. For, as previously explained, the obvious side effects of drugs may "break the blind" and allow participants and doctors to determine which is a drug and which is placebo.

Besides helping individuals know whether they are taking drugs or placebo, side effects throw another monkey wrench into the works by turning drugs into "active placebos." This term refers to the following phenomenon: When a drug produces demonstrable symptoms, even unpleasant ones, its ordinary power of suggestion may be enhanced. You might say, "Since I have a dry mouth and my heart is racing, I know I'm taking a powerful drug." Some authorities have recommended using drugs such as antihistamines instead of sugar pills for placebo, to balance out this particular form of the placebo effect.

However, St. John's wort has a strike against it in this regard: It's so gentle, you might come to the conclusion that it can't possibly be doing anything. This is precisely what happened in the case of my patient Laura, described earlier. Laura was absolutely certain St. John's wort couldn't be working for her because she didn't feel lousy when she took it! This impression actively blocked her awareness of its genuine effects.

Thus the power of suggestion may be confounding our evaluation of the relative effectiveness of St. John's wort versus chemical antidepressants. Research carefully designed to eliminate this problem may demonstrate that St. John's wort is actually just as powerful for mild to moderate depression as any drug—*if* the uneven effects of suggestion are removed.

Side-Effect Comparison

In almost all studies of St. John's wort, the incidence of side effects is extremely low. As described in the last chapter, one trial of 3,250 individuals given St. John's wort showed a total side-effect rate of only 2.4%.[12] The most common reported problem was stomach distress (0.6%), followed by allergic reactions (0.5%) and tiredness (0.4%).

This large study was not blinded. When all the double-blind trials comparing St. John's wort to placebo are lumped together, the observed incidence of side effects attributed to St. John's wort is 4.1%.[13] This is still far lower than the incidence of side effects attributable to antidepressant drugs.

Tricyclic antidepressants produce side effects in virtually everyone who takes them. The newer antidepressants are better, but they are still far more prone to side effects than St. John's wort. According to the 1997 *PDR*, 10 to 15% of people taking Prozac develop so much anxiety, nervousness, or insomnia that they are compelled to quit taking the drug. The incidence of sexual side effects may be as high as 30% or more.[14] One German study showed an overall Prozac side-effect rate of approximately 19%, which is about five to eight times greater than the occurrence rate with St. John's wort.[15] This particular figure may be especially meaningful because, like the St. John's wort studies cited, it involved German observers and participants and thus compares apples to apples.

Another way to look at the question is to examine the rate at which people discontinue medications due to adverse effects. Approximately 31% of individuals given tricyclic antidepressants quit taking them because of side effects.[16] The numbers with Prozac seem to be somewhat lower, perhaps around 17%,[17] although the exact number remains a matter of controversy. In comparison, only 1.5% of those taking St. John's wort discontinue due to side effects, according to the 3,250-participant drug-monitoring study just mentioned in the preceding text.

These differences in side effects make a compelling case for trying St. John's wort before conventional drugs.

An Interesting Discrepancy

The St. John's wort side-effects figures cited previously were derived from the combined results of the 3,250 participant drug-monitoring study and the St. John's wort versus placebo studies. Nevertheless, a few studies report much higher percentages of side effects. The origin of these inconsistent results demonstrates yet another fascinating example of the placebo effect.

In the St. John's wort versus imipramine study discussed earlier, a full 12% of the individuals taking St. John's wort reported side effects, the most frequent being dry mouth and dizziness.[18] This is three times or more the total incidence of side effects reported in other studies, and remarkably close to the 16% of participants who developed side effects on low doses of imipramine. It is important to note as well that dry mouth and dizziness were also the predominating imipramine side effects.

Another significant fact is that while the numbers were close, the perceived intensity of side effects was quite different in those taking the herb versus those taking the drug. Nearly all individuals on St. John's wort said their side effects were mild, while for those on the low doses of imipramine, 7 out of 22 participants complained of moderate to severe side effects.

Nonetheless, one may ask why these side effects for St. John's wort occurred at all. Dry mouth was not even an issue in the trial of 3,250 participants, and dizziness occurred at a very low rate of 0.15%. Why should dry mouth and dizziness suddenly show up in high percentages when St. John's wort is being compared to imipramine? This bizarre change deserves an explanation.

Fortunately, it's not hard to find one. Imipramine is a drug famous for causing dry mouth and dizziness. When taken in full doses, it causes dry mouth in virtually all people and dizziness in a high percentage. What we are probably seeing here is a kind of shadow effect caused by suggestion. Participants in a double-blind comparison between drug and herb *think* they may be taking a drug and thus develop some of the side effects they expect from the drug—even when they're not taking it.

A confirmation of this explanation may be found in drug versus placebo studies. Those given placebo typically develop side effects at remarkable levels when they think they may be taking a real drug. For example, in the Zoloft-imipramine-placebo study cited earlier, 17% of the participants taking placebo reported dry mouth and 16%

reported dizziness.[19] The same kind of shadow effect is at work here.

Thus the high rates of side effects seen in St. John's wort versus drug tests are probably falsely inflated. The 2.4 to 4.1% rate discovered in all other studies is much more likely to be correct.

Safety Issues

Side effects and safety are slightly different issues. One refers to annoying problems, the other to the risks of serious injury or even death. For example, MAO inhibitors may give you insomnia as a side effect, but if you eat the wrong foods while taking them you might die. Similarly, tricyclic drugs will almost certainly make your mouth dry. However, if you accidentally take as little as four times the recommended amount, you may end up in the hospital with seizures, heart injury, dangerously low blood pressure, or even coma. Many depressed individuals taking prescribed tricyclics have used them to commit suicide.

The Prozac family of drugs is far safer than either MAO inhibitors or tricyclics. Individuals have taken as much as 100 tablets at a time with no worse result than agitation and vomiting (although there have been a few reports of more serious injury). This safety factor figured extensively in Prozac's early advertising campaign. As one drug representative said in recommendation of his product, "Even if it doesn't work, your patient won't be able to kill himself with it."

St. John's wort is also quite safe. Although many millions of people have taken it in Germany, no serious adverse effects have been recorded. Studies involving physical exam and serial blood tests have never shown any measurable effects.[20] Photosensitivity and MAO inhibitor–like side effects are sometimes mentioned as risks; but, as discussed in the previous chapter, the latter probably does not exist at all and the former only occurs occasionally with doses higher than normally prescribed.

Nevertheless, firm statements about long-term safety cannot be made for either St. John's wort or any pharmaceutical antidepressant. In chapter 4, I explained how such a determination would require difficult studies that would take many years. I also described a particular concern regarding Prozac: It may cause long-term injury analogous to tardive dyskinesia, the distressing and permanent movement disorder that occurs in some people who take antischizophrenic drugs.

While this risk remains speculative, Scott Shannon thinks that it is a realistic enough basis for limiting the use of Prozac in mild to moderate depression. "I think we need to be very careful about prescribing drugs that dramatically change brain chemicals," he says. "We don't really know all the ramifications. I wouldn't like to give Prozac to someone with mild to moderate depression and find out later that I've caused some kind of long-term harm."

Of course, it is possible that St. John's wort could cause long-term harm as well. As mentioned in the last chapter, there's no way to know.

Psychological "Side Effects"

Another safety issue with regard to use of antidepressants refers to psychological rather than physical risks. This type of potential harm from using Prozac and other antidepressant drugs is seldom mentioned, but may pose a danger as serious in its own way as outright chemical toxicity.

Those who depend on Prozac for psychological well-being may experience a subtle but damaging distortion of self-image. "I need drugs to be normal," goes the unspoken refrain, and it is a damaging message that may cause real harm. Children who are taking Prozac may be the

Let's Be Fair, Part II

Just as news media and medical authorities tend to criticize natural treatments unfairly, proponents of alternative medicine frequently do the same to conventional treatments. Prozac is a frequent victim of this form of exaggeration. It has been demonized as a deadly drug causing suicide, murder, and violent agitation.

Actually, Prozac is quite safe as far as drugs go, much safer, in fact, than numerous common over-the-counter drugs. My suggestion? Let's tone down the rhetoric, and talk about both drugs and natural treatments fairly.

most susceptible to this subtle harm because their developing identities may permanently incorporate this sense of dependence on an artificial substance.

In contrast, St. John's wort gives a completely different and far more wholesome message. Psychologically speaking, it "feels" more like a food than a drug; it's a natural plant rather than a synthetic chemical. This emotional point is usually disregarded by physicians who have difficulty recognizing the problem because their profession makes them perfectly comfortable with drugs.

Increasingly, Prozac has been offered as a treatment for mildly depressed children. But, considering this point, I question whether it is always worth the risk. Chronic dependency on a drug may do psychological damage that outweighs the good produced by relief of depression. If there were no other choice but to use Prozac, physicians and parents might deem that risk warranted. However, since St. John's wort represents an effective and more psychologically wholesome alternative, it may be a preferable option. (Please note that neither Prozac nor St. John's wort has been fully evaluated for its benefit in treating children, although Prozac's manufacturer was nearing completion of the process to approve its use in children at press time.)

Does St. John's Wort Produce Exactly the Same Effects on Depression As Antidepressant Drugs?

There is still one more level of comparison between St. John's wort and drug antidepressants to consider. Amidst all the HAM-D values and formal evaluation criteria, the inward nature of depression, and recovery from it, includes many indefinable experiences that could be significant. Emotional suffering is beyond the crude grasp of rating scales. It would be like trying to measure the extent of good character or the depth of gratitude.

This is an area that eludes science and moves into the realm of literature and poetry. A writer might fill hundreds of pages detailing a person's inner life and still fail to capture it completely, so you can see that a 17-item HAM-D can't possibly come close.

It is for this reason that, even when two antidepressants produce similarly measured changes in depression, their actual effects may be quite different. Peter Kramer speaks of different layers, or levels, of depression, some of which tricyclic drugs seem to "touch," others of which seem more accessible to Prozac. St. John's wort may touch areas of the mind unique to itself.

Actually, each antidepressant drug probably produces its own characteristic effects on depression; and if language could easily describe such differences, more people would talk about it. The best descriptions I've heard came from two unusually expressive individuals. Their excellent communication skills have given me a glimpse of these largely unrecognized distinctions.

"Prozac turns on an 'outgoing' button in me," says Caroline, a 40-year-old freelance writer. "I find myself talking to people in a more assertive, pushy way, almost without even noticing. It's as if Prozac pushes a switch and turns me into an extrovert. I like feeling less depressed, but I don't always want to feel the way Prozac wants me to feel."

Caroline has tried other antidepressants, too, and rates them differently. "Wellbutrin doesn't push the extrovert button. Instead it turns up the 'contrast' dial, increasing my mental clarity. I can think more clearly, organize myself better, and get more things done. I become an effective workaholic instead of an aggressive party animal. On Wellbutrin, I *like* cleaning house, which says a lot. However, my feelings seem shoved way in the background."

She's also taken Serzone. "Now that's a really different medication. It makes me moody and dreamy and languid. The moods are happy and the dreams are interesting. However, I feel so dreamy that I don't talk to people or get anything done."

Caroline puts St. John's wort in its own class. "What St. John's wort does for me is to put me in a bouncy mood, what they used to call a 'sanguine' disposition. I feel carefree, light, and even a bit euphoric. It doesn't make me as assertive as Prozac, as organized as Wellbutrin, nor as dreamy as Serzone, but it feels more normal."

Another individuals, whom I shall call Jim, says that he finds Prozac very gentle. "It doesn't give me any side effects," says this 56-year-old civil servant. "All I notice when I take it is that I don't waste my time second-guessing myself. I make my decisions and carry them through without obsessing over them. I feel more myself on Prozac."

But Jim appreciates St. John's wort, as well. "I also feel more myself on St. John's wort but it's a different 'self.' The herb doesn't stop me from chewing things over in my mind, like Prozac does, but it does stop me from getting tied up in knots about it. You could put it this way: Prozac turns me into a shoot-from-the-hip, John Wayne kind of guy, while St. John's wort makes me more like Gregory Peck. You know, the calm, reflective type. I'm not sure which I like best."

This type of thoughtful analysis belongs to a larger discussion about the nature of personality and the appropriateness or inappropriateness of using substances to modify it. Certainly, there is no reason to believe that anyone else will experience antidepressant treatments in exactly the same ways that Caroline or Jim does. My purpose in mentioning their descriptions is not to dictate how you'll feel, but simply to show that there are many personal details that must be taken into account.

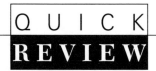

QUICK REVIEW

- Unfortunately, due to flaws in the scientific studies, we can't say for certain how St. John's wort compares to conventional treatment. However, based on the evidence we do have, the herb appears to be approximately as effective for mild to moderate depression.

- St. John's wort is probably less effective in treating severe depression.
- St. John's wort clearly produces fewer side effects on average than conventional treatments for depression.

Other Alternative Treatments for Depression

Alternative medicine is an immense field, almost a world unto itself. While some approaches within this world are ridiculous, others are reasonably practical, and a few are nearly as scientific as most conventional treatments. This complex subject is discussed in greater detail in my book *The Alternative Medicine Sourcebook: A Realistic Evaluation of Alternative Healing Options* (Lowell House, 1997).

None of the techniques described in this chapter have been as solidly researched (with regard to their effects in treating depression) as St. John's wort. However, most have some research backing, and all seem to work at least occasionally. Alternative practitioners frequently combine these methods with St. John's wort to increase its effect. However, the safety of such combinations is unknown. They can also be tried as a substitute for St. John's wort when the herb fails to produce satisfactory results.

Ginkgo Biloba: Improving Mental Function

The ginkgo biloba tree is a beautiful ornamental that can grow more than 100 feet tall and live for longer than 1,000 years (see figure 3). It has been called "the living fossil" because evidence of its existence can be traced back more than 200 million years. Once distributed on many continents, it was nearly wiped out during the Ice Ages and survived only in China. However, the resilience it developed during its long tenure on earth has given it the power to survive a new hostile environment: that of modern city streets. Because of its superb resistance to insects, disease, and air pollution ginkgo has become a widely planted sidewalk decoration.

The medicinal use of ginkgo goes back to ancient China, where its fruit was used as a standard part of the extensive Chinese medical repertoire. Its traditional uses included "benefiting the brain," as well as aiding respiratory illnesses and ridding the body of parasitic worms.

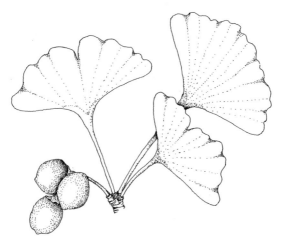

Figure 3. *Ginkgo*

What Is Ginkgo Used for Today?

In modern times standardized extracts of the ginkgo leaf have been extensively researched in Europe. Most of the research into ginkgo has concentrated on its ability to improve mental function in the elderly. Ginkgo is also prescribed for intermittent claudication, the pain with exercise that occurs when arteries are blocked by atherosclerotic changes. According to the respected naturopath Michael Murray, ginkgo extract accounts for 1.5% of all prescription sales in France and 1% of those in Germany.[1]

What Is the Scientific Evidence?

During the studies on impaired mental functions, researchers frequently observed improvements in mood and relief from symptoms of depression. This incidental discovery led scientists to investigate whether ginkgo might be useful as an antidepressant treatment. One study published in 1990 evaluated this effect in 60 inpatients who suffered from depressive symptoms along with other signs of dementia.[2] The results showed significant improvements among those given ginkgo extract instead of placebo.

Another study followed 40 depressed individuals over the age of 50 who had not responded successfully to antidepressant treatment.[3] Those who were given ginkgo showed an average drop in HAM-D scores of 50%, while the placebo group showed only a 10% improvement.

In 1994 an interesting piece of research was reported that may shed light on the mechanism by which ginkgo could improve depression.[4] This study examined levels of serotonin receptors in rats of various ages. When older rats were given ginkgo, the level of serotonin binding sites increased. The same effect was *not* observed, however, in younger rats. The researchers theorized that ginkgo may block an age-related loss of serotonin receptors.

Reduced receptors for serotonin may mean that the body needs more serotonin to produce a normal effect.

Marilyn's Story

In my own practice, I've seen many individuals who reported significant improvement through taking ginkgo extract. One of the most dramatic cases is Marilyn, a woman who, in her late sixties, had become morose and withdrawn. Fearing Alzheimer's disease, her daughter had given Marilyn ginkgo, hoping it would improve her mental functioning. The results were impressive. In about 3 weeks, Marilyn was back to macramé, letter writing, and going for long walks with her friends.

She continued this way for 1 year. Then, due to the expense, Marilyn stopped taking ginkgo. Within 1 month she was living in her recliner again.

A subsequent medical evaluation showed that Marilyn didn't have Alzheimer's. She was merely depressed. Her physician then prescribed Prozac, with excellent results. However, ginkgo had worked just as well. In this case the natural treatment was just as effective as the drug.

Instead of raising the level of serotonin, like Prozac, ginkgo may thus improve the brain's ability to respond to serotonin (at least in older people). But this is still highly speculative. More experimentation is needed to clarify the mechanism of ginkgo's action and to better quantify its effectiveness in treating depression.

Dosage

The proper dose is 40 to 80 mg 3 times daily of a 50:1 extract standardized to contain 24% ginkgo flavonoid glycosides (heterosides) and 6% terpene lactones. It may take 2 to 8 weeks for the full effect to develop. Ginkgo is expensive, ranging from $20 to $50 per month.

Safety Issues

Ginkgo leaf extract appears to be quite safe. (Ginkgo fruit and seeds are definitely toxic, but they are not used in the United States.) Among 9,722 individuals who were given standard ginkgo formulations in double-blind studies, the most common side effect was mild stomach discomfort; and this only occurred in about 0.2% of the studied participants.[5] Headaches and dizziness were the next most common problems. In animal studies gigantic doses of ginkgo extract are required before fatalities occur. However, there have been some case reports of abnormal bleeding in those who combined ginkgo and blood-thinning drugs. It has not been proven that ginkgo was really at fault, but to be on the safe side, if you are taking a blood-thinning medication, you should definitely discuss the subject with your doctor prior to taking ginkgo. It is also remotely possible that combining gingko with natural substances that mildly thin the blood could also cause problems, including garlic, phosphatidylserine, and high-dose vitamin E.

Safety for young children, pregnant or nursing women, and those with liver or kidney disease has not been established. (For more information, see *The Natural Pharmacist Guide to Ginkgo and Memory.*)

Phenylalanine (DLPA): The Amino Acid Antidepressant

Phenylalanine is a naturally occurring amino acid that we all consume in our daily diets. Artificial supplementation with phenylalanine seems sometimes to be effective in the treatment of depression. Many alternative practitioners use it along with St. John's wort and report enhanced results.

Randy's Story

Numerous individuals have told me DLPA helped them. One such was a 32-year-old salesman named Randy, who had found himself increasingly unmotivated at work. He enjoyed his job and was successful at it, but he was finding it increasingly difficult to keep his focus. "It's not like me," he would say. "I feel so gloomy when I get to work."

I suggested that he might be subconsciously interested in changing his career, but he adamantly opposed that theory. "The job's great," he said. "The people are great, I believe in my product, and the money's good. This depression is coming out of nowhere."

Because I wouldn't stop suggesting psychological angles, Randy finally quit seeing me and visited a naturopath instead.

The body can convert phenylalanine into a variety of biological amines. While this may eventually explain its apparent antidepressant effects, what is known thus far about its mechanism of action can only be regarded as highly preliminary and speculative. The evidence for its effectiveness also remains preliminary.

What Is the Scientific Evidence for Phenylalanine?

Like many other chemicals in the body, phenylalanine exists in two forms that are mirror images of each other. These two forms are known as D- and L-phenylalanine. Some studies have evaluated the D form, and others the L form, while still others evaluated mixtures of both. The mixed DL form (DLPA) is the product most commonly available in stores.

A 1978 study compared the effectiveness of D-phenylalanine against the antidepressant drug imipramine, given

I didn't hear from him for 3 months. Then he called to let me know what had worked, and even before he told me anything about the treatment I was already impressed by how good he sounded.

"I started taking DL-phenylalanine about a month ago. The stuff's incredible. I don't even remember what it feels like to be depressed."

His voice was sparkling and full of life. When I asked him what he had tried the first 2 months, he said, "First she put me on some kind of wort. John's wort, or something like that. It didn't do a thing. But this DL-phenylalanine, it's powerful." However, anecdotes such as this one don't prove anything. More research is needed.

in the somewhat low (but probably effective) dose of 100 mg daily.[6] A total of 60 patients were randomly assigned to either one group or the other and followed for 30 days. The results in both groups were statistically equivalent. However, D-phenylalanine worked more rapidly, producing significant improvement in only 15 days.

Another double-blind study followed 27 individuals, half of whom received DL-phenylalanine and the other half imipramine in full doses of 150 to 200 mg.[7] When they were reevaluated in 30 days, the two groups had improved by the same statistical margin.

I have been unable to find any halfway decent studies that directly compared phenylalanine to placebo. Several such studies have been performed, but they were all either far too small or too flawed to be worth reporting. Much more research needs to be done before phenylalanine can be considered a proven treatment for depression. Nonetheless, phenylalanine certainly appears to be effective in practice. I recently surveyed a panel of expert alternative practitioners in order to provide the data for the *Alternative Medicine Ratings Guide* (Prima, 1998). DL-phenylalanine was one of the most popular antidepressant treatments, rated at a level of "often effective."

Dosage

In clinical practice, most physicians prescribe from 150 to 400 mg daily of DL-phenylalanine, divided up into 2 or 3 daily doses.

Safety Issues

Phenylalanine is believed to be safe, although comprehensive safety studies have not been performed. Side effects are rare, although increased anxiety, headache, and even mild hypertension have been occasionally reported when higher doses of phenylalanine were used. Phenylalanine must be avoided by those with the rare metabolic disease phenylketonuria (PKU). Safety for young children, pregnant or nursing women, and those with liver or kidney disease has not been established.

5-HTP: One Step
Away from Serotonin

A new, up-and-coming treatment for depression is 5-hydroxy-tryptophan, or 5-HTP for short. When the body sets about manufacturing serotonin, it first makes 5-HTP. The theory behind using 5-HTP as a supplement is that providing the raw ingredient that's just one step back from serotonin might induce the body to manufacture more serotonin on its own. However, this reasonable guess has not been proven.

Like St. John's wort, 5-HTP is primarily used in Europe, where many physicians consider it an effective treatment for both depression and insomnia. Recent questions about safety have put a damper on enthusiasm for this treatment (see following section on safety issues).

What Is the Scientific Evidence?

Unfortunately, the scientific evidence for 5-HTP is not strong. The best study was a 6-week trial of 63 people given either 5-HTP or full doses of the European antidepressant Luvox (a drug similar to Prozac).[8] Overall, 5-HTP produced the same antidepressant benefits as Luvox, with fewer and less severe side effects. However, this was a small study. More and better research is necessary to determine whether 5-HTP is really effective as an antidepressant.

More experimentation is needed to clarify the mechanism of ginkgo's action and to better quantify its effectiveness in treating depression.

Dosage

The typical dose of 5-HTP is 100 to 200 mg 3 times daily.

Safety Issues

In general, 5-HTP appears to be safe when used as directed. Side effects appear to be limited to the usual occasional mild digestive distress and allergic reactions. However, an unexpected safety concern has raised questions about the use of this supplement. To explain it, I must first step back and talk about the amino acid tryptophan.

Tryptophan used to be recommended as a treatment for depression on a similar basis as 5-HTP, because it is one step back in the chain (the body turns tryptophan into 5-HTP and the 5-HTP is then turned into serotonin). However, tryptophan was removed from the stores several years ago when a contaminant caused a terrible, often permanently disabling and sometimes even fatal illness in many people who took the supplement.

Because 5-HTP is made by a completely different manufacturing process (starting from a plant rather than a bacteria), you would not expect there to be any risk of the same contaminant appearing. Surprisingly, however, in September of 1998, the FDA released a report stating that some commercial 5-HTP preparations might contain the same contaminant as tryptophan. Because this is late-breaking news, I suggest you check with your physician for the most recent information.

Much more research needs to be done before phenylalanine can be considered a proven treatment for depression.

Safety for young children, pregnant or nursing mothers, or those with liver or kidney disease has not been established.

SAMe: Expensive but May Work Rapidly

Another European supplement treatment for depression recently introduced in the United States is S-adenosylmethionine, or SAMe for short. SAMe is a very important biological molecule that occurs throughout the body. Its job is to hand over a chemical fragment called a methyl group to other chemicals that need it. SAMe is particularly popular in Italy, where some physicians report that it is an especially rapidly acting antidepressant. They sometimes use SAMe alongside conventional antidepressants at the very beginning of treatment to provide immediate relief. SAMe is also used as a treatment for osteoarthritis, for which it has a moderately strong research record. Unfortunately, the sum total of evidence for SAMe as an antidepressant remains small and flawed by the fact that most studies used an intravenous form of the supplement.

Besides a lack of reliable evidence, SAMe is extremely expensive. The proper dose is 400 mg 4 times a day, which can cost over $200 per month. Hopefully, the price will come down as SAMe becomes more widely accepted. Most physicians recommend starting at a low dose of perhaps 200 mg twice a day, and then gradually working up, to minimize stomach distress. Once you reach the full dose, stay at it for 1 month or so. If you start feeling better, you can try reducing the dose. Some physicians report that as low a dose as 400 mg a day may be effective for maintaining antidepressant benefits.

SAMe appears to be a nontoxic substance. However, safety for young children, pregnant or nursing women, and those with liver or kidney disease has not been established.

Phosphatidylserine: A Supplement That Works Like Ginkgo

Phosphatidylserine is one of the chemicals that the body uses to maintain the integrity of cell membranes, and it is the primary such chemical used in the brain.[9] It is not an essential nutrient because cells can manufacture this substance themselves. However, when taken as a food supplement phosphatidylserine sometimes seems to improve brain function.

Most of the research on this chemical has concentrated on elderly patients with mental impairment. One double-blind study followed 494 individuals with Alzheimer's-like symptoms for 6 months, and the results demonstrated that phosphatidylserine improved mental function, mood, and behavior.[10] So far, only one study has concentrated on this substance's effectiveness in depression.[11] The results appear to be favorable, but further research needs to be done.

In actual clinical practice, I have rarely heard of anyone whose depression was cured simply by taking a multivitamin, however, supplementation may still be helpful as a supportive treatment.

In clinical practice, physicians who use phosphatidylserine report marked improvement in some depressed individuals over 50. It seems to be most beneficial in those for whom mental decline is an important part of the picture.

The proper dose of phosphatidylserine is 100 mg 3 times daily. Full results take anywhere from 4 weeks to 6 months to manifest. Although there do not seem to be any side effects, this is a very expensive supplement, usually costing in the range of $50 to $75 per month. As with gingko, caution is necessary when combining phsophatidylserine with blood-thinning drugs, and there are theoretical concerns regarding combining it with natural blood thinners such as garlic, gingko, and vitamin E. Safety for young children, pregnant or nursing women, and those with liver or kidney disease has not been established.

Nutrient Deficiencies

Contrary to what you might read, treatment with phenylalanine, 5-HTP, SAMe, or phosphatidylserine should not really be considered nutritional medicine. Most Americans receive satisfactory amounts of phenylalanine in their daily diet, and 5-HTP, SAMe, and phosphatidylserine are not normally consumed in significant quantities at all.

A true nutritional treatment corrects a dietary deficiency. Depression can be a symptom of inadequate intake of folic acid, vitamin B_6, vitamin B_{12}, magnesium, iron, or essential fatty acids. Because studies have shown widespread deficiencies in some of these common nutrients,[12] it is reasonable to assume that in some cases of depression simple supplementation may make a difference.

Fatty acids are an exception to this rule. These nutrients can be easily supplemented through standard vitamin and mineral pills. However, don't take iron supplements unless you know that you are deficient. The best source of "good" essential fatty acids is probably cold-water fish, but flax oil, taken at a dose of 1 or 2 tablespoons a day, may be useful as well.

Despite the logic behind such supplementation, in actual clinical practice I have rarely heard of anyone whose depression was cured simply by taking a multivitamin. It seems that while severe deficiency of common nutrients can certainly cause depression, slight deficiencies rarely produce noticeable effects. However, supplementation may still be helpful as a supportive treatment.

Lifestyle Changes

Thus far, this chapter has primarily focused on treatment options for depression that consist of specific, targeted methods. These approaches are the easiest to use and evaluate, but by concentrating on them I've invited fierce criticism from my colleagues in alternative medicine. "We're supposed to treat the whole person," they say to me, and I have to agree.

The best approach to any illness is a holistic one that involves many dimensions of the self. I've previously stressed the importance of psychotherapy, but it may also be essential to consider the impact of lifestyle factors. In the clinic, I always ask questions such as: Do you exercise? What's your stress level? Do you have a good diet? And do you enjoy your job, your social life, and your living situation?

If you don't take care of yourself as a whole person, it's quite possible that more specific treatments will fail to work. Probably the simplest lifestyle change is to increase your exercise level. Numerous clinical studies seem to indicate that exercise is an effective antidepressant. While other studies contradict this intuitive result, the least that can be said is that it won't cause you any harm. Exercise increases overall health and energy, reduces the risk of many illnesses, and relieves stress.

Speaking of stress, there is no question that excessive stress can put most anyone into a depression. Although life is inevitably full of stresses, there are numerous activities that can moderate their impact. Some of the most useful include regular exercise, meditation, prayer, good social interactions, play, visualizations, regular massage, and extended vacations.

It is also important to consider the effects of overall diet. Psychoactive substances such as caffeine, alcohol, and even chocolate may lead to increased depression in many people. Other substances, such as sugar and fat, can also increase depression in a few individuals. As previously mentioned, dietary deficiencies of important nutrients may sometimes play a role in depression as well. Good diet, like regular exercise, provides numerous health benefits, so it certainly fits into the "couldn't hurt" category.

Finally, depression can be caused by life choices and situations. If you are in an abusive marriage, if you hate your job, or if you have no friends, depression is a likely result. An excessive focus on status and money and not enough on love can also make you miserable. This last subject is the topic of innumerable plays, movies, and books—not to mention religious scripture—and it has never stopped being true.

I remember a man in his 40s who came to me when Prozac failed to alleviate his depression. His life was devoted solely to pursuing a higher standing in the state bureaucracy of Washington. My first impression was that he was miserable because his priorities were confused. Never did he spend more than 2 hours a week with his children, although he bought them expensive presents, and his primary idea of a good time seemed to be buttering up superiors and scheming against competitors. For recreation, he watched the news and ate hamburgers.

In clinical practice kava is usually not as potent as standard drugs for anxiety. Its good side-effects profile, however, may make it worth trying first.

I prescribed St. John's wort, but it didn't do him any good. He needed to make other positive lifestyle changes. Unfortunately, it took 2 years and a heart attack to put things in perspective for him. Fortunately, this catastrophe opened his eyes, and he actually began to institute major changes in his life. Luckily, his heart wasn't badly damaged, and he now has a good chance of living a more satisfying life for many years to come.

As this man found, changing deeply embedded life patterns can be quite difficult. Nevertheless, there are ways to accomplish it without nearly dying. Friends, counselors, clergy, social workers, and physicians all may be able to assist you in initiating positive changes. Sometimes the boost of an antidepressant (whether herbal or pharmaceutical) may also be useful as a kind of "jump-start."

Supplemental Treatments for Anxiety

Anxiety frequently accompanies depression. While relief from anxiety symptoms may result from taking St. John's wort, it may only be after the herb's full effect develops in 4 to 6 weeks. Sometimes a more rapidly acting treatment is needed. Conventional medicine uses a group of drugs called anxiolytics for this purpose. Alternative medicine has at least a couple of good options that can be tried as well. However, if you suffer from severe anxiety, make sure to seek medical attention. It is also important to rule out underlying medical diseases, such as hyperthyroidism, that can cause anxiety symptoms.

European physicians frequently use the root of the *Piper methysticum* plant, commonly known as kava, as a short-term treatment for anxiety. This member of the pepper family has long been cultivated by Pacific islanders (see figure 4). They make a drink out of kava and consume it on ceremonial occasions. In small doses, this drink produces relaxation, while larger doses induce sleep.

Standardized extracts of kava have been approved in Germany and other European countries for the treatment of anxiety and insomnia. Several double-blind studies document kava's effectiveness. For example, one study followed 100 individuals with anxiety, half of whom received kava extract and the other half placebo.[13] Over the course of the 6-month trial, the Hamilton Anxiety scale (analogous to the HAM-D scale used for depression) was administered to rate the level of anxiety. The HAM-A quantifies symptoms such as restlessness, nervousness, heart palpitations, stomach discomfort, dizziness, and chest pain. Participants given kava instead of placebo showed dramatically better results than those on placebo, but without significant side effects.

While a double dose of oxazepam impairs alertness, a double dose of kava does not adversely affect alertness.[14]

In clinical practice kava is usually not as potent as standard drugs for anxiety. Its good side-effects profile, however, may make it worth trying first. A typical dose should be standardized on the basis of kavalactone content and

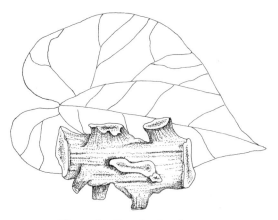

Figure 4. *Kava leaf and root*

taken to provide 60 to 210 mg of kavalactones daily, divided up in 3 doses. Please note that safety of kava–St. John's wort combination treatment has not been proven.

Research suggests that kava's antianxiety effects begin within 1 week and continue to increase over an additional 2 weeks. At standard doses, kava does not generally cause any side effects. A few reports indicate that it may occasionally produce symptoms reminiscent of Parkinson's disease, however, so it is not recommended for those with that illness. Ten times the normal dose can cause a particular skin rash known as *kava dermopathy*. Even larger doses may cause a variety of changes on lab tests, although those people in whom this effect has been observed were also alcoholics, making any conclusions suspect.[15]

Kava should not be combined with other sedatives, because the effects may add up, producing too much sedation. There have been reports of coma induced by the combination of kava and standard tranquilizers. As mentioned, it is also not clear whether it's safe to combine kava with St. John's wort. Safety for young children, pregnant or nursing women, and those with liver or kidney disease has not been established. (For more information, see *The Natural Pharmacist Guide to Kava and Anxiety.*)

Besides kava, there are also a number of European herbs traditionally used for anxiety, including hops, lady's slipper, skullcap, lobelia, and rauwolfia. However, the effects of these other herbs seem to be rather mild, yet at the same time they may present real dangers if used in excessive doses.

Kava should not be combined with other sedatives, because the effects may add up, producing too much sedation.

Other possibly useful treatments for anxiety include calcium (1,000 mg a day), magnesium (500 mg a day), and vitamin B_6 (50 mg a day). These food supplements may be particularly effective in treating anxiety associated with PMS.

Supplemental Treatments for Insomnia

Insomnia is another symptom that commonly goes along with depression. Just as for anxiety, there are a number of alternative treatments that may be useful while waiting for St. John's wort to kick in. However, please note that safety when combined with St. John's wort has not been established.

Small-sized double-blind studies suggest that the herb valerian is significantly more effective than placebo, without producing morning sleepiness.[16] Valerian's benefits for insomnia also occur without the side effects of daytime drowsiness or disturbances of sleep stages. In clinical practice valerian is seldom as powerful as pharmaceutical sleeping pills and it may take many weeks of use to achieve full effects. The proper dose of valerian is 1 to 2 g of dried root, or

150 to 300 mg of valerian extract standardized to 0.8% valeric acid. It should be taken 20 minutes before bedtime. Do not combine valerian with other sedative drugs or drive within 2 hours of taking it. While valerian is generally regarded as safe, it has a highly unpleasant odor. Safety for young children, pregnant or nursing women, and those with liver or kidney disease has not been established.

Kava is another possible option for insomnia, taken at a dose of 200 to 300 mg 1 hour before bed. Other herbs used for insomnia include hops, passionflower, lady's slipper, skullcap, and lobelia. These herbs appear to be less effective than kava or valerian, however, and some can be dangerous if taken to excess.

Finally, visualization tapes, meditation, and yoga may make falling asleep easier and even improve sleep quality.

Valerian's benefits for insomnia occur without the side effects of morning sleepiness, daytime drowsiness, or disturbances of sleep stages. However, it's seldom as powerful as pharmaceutical sleeping pills.

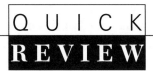

QUICK REVIEW

- **Although St. John's wort can be helpful in depression, it doesn't always work. Besides turning to conventional medications, there are also a number of other natural therapies** you could try. However, none of them has as much research evidence behind it as St. John's wort.

- Ginkgo (40 mg 3 times daily of a 50:1 extract standardized to 24% gingko flavonoid glycosides and 6% terpene lactones) and phosphatidylserine (100 mg 3 times daily) may be helpful for depression in those over 50 years of age. Gingko should not be combined with blood-thinning drugs such as Coumadin (warfarin), heparin, or even aspirin, except on the advice of a physician. It is also remotely possible that combining gingko with natural substances that mildly thin the blood could also cause problems, including garlic, phosphatidylserine, and high-dose vitamin E. As with gingko, caution is necessary when combining phosphatidylerine with blood-thinning drugs, and there are theoretical concerns regarding combining it with natural blood thinners such as garlic, gingko, and high-dose vitamin E.

- DL-phenylalanine, 5-HTP, and S-adenosylmethionine may be helpful in other age groups as well.

- Nutritional supplementation with folic acid, vitamin B_6, vitamin B_{12}, magnesium, iron, and essential fatty acids may help if your diet leaves you deficient in these nutrients.

- When depression is accompanied by insomnia or anxiety the herbs kava (20 to 70 mg of kavalactones 3 times daily) and valerian (1 to 2 g of dried root or 150 to 300 mg of extract standardized to 0.8% valeric acid 20 minutes before bedtime) may offer additional benefit. Do not combine valerian with other sedative drugs or drive within 2 hours of taking it. However, we do not know whether it is safe to combine kava or valerian with St. John's wort.

- Lifestyle changes are important and shouldn't be neglected. Diet, exercise, and other lifestyle choices may play a significant role in the state of your mood.

Putting It All Together

For your easy reference, this chapter contains a brief summary of key information contained in this book. Please refer to earlier chapters for more comprehensive information, including a detailed discussion of safety issues.

St. John's wort is one of the best documented of all herbal treatments. Double-blind studies involving a total of nearly 900 individuals suggest that it is an effective treatment for mild to moderate depression. In Germany, prescriptions for St. John's wort are covered by the national health-care system, and it is prescribed more frequently than any synthetic antidepressant drug in that country.

However, St. John's wort is not effective for severe depression. **Warning:** I strongly recommend getting a physician's evaluation before self-treating with this herb, because it is possible to be dangerously depressed without knowing it. Also, other medical illnesses can masquerade as depression. However, if your physician does determine that you suffer from mild to moderate depression, St. John's wort may be your best option.

St. John's wort appears to be effective in about 55% of cases. The big potential advantage of St. John's wort over standard medications is that it rarely, if ever, causes side effects. As with any herb or drug, allergic reactions are possible, and some people develop mild digestive distress.

The proper dose of St. John's wort is 300 mg 3 times daily (or 600 mg in the morning and 300 mg in the evening) of a dose standardized to contain 0.3% hypericin. New products may be standardized to 3 to 5% hyperiform. If the herb bothers your stomach, take it with food. As with other antidepressants, the full effect takes approximately 4 to 6 weeks to develop, so be patient.

St. John's wort appears to be very safe. However, if highly sun-sensitive people take more than the normal dose of the herb, they may sunburn more quickly. To be on the safe side, if you're especially sensitive to the sun, don't exceed the recommended dose of St. John's wort and continue to take your usual precautions against sunburns.

Older reports suggested that St. John's wort works like the class of drugs known as MAO inhibitors. This led to a number of warnings, including avoiding cheese and decongestants while taking St. John's wort. However, this concern is no longer considered realistic.

It may not be safe to combine St. John's wort with other antidepressant drugs. Because Prozac stays in the system for quite a while, you should consult a physician if you want to make a transition from Prozac to St. John's wort.

It has also been suggested that St. John's wort may interact with drugs that are metabolized by cytochrome P-450 CYP 1A1 and 1A2. Ask your physician if you are taking any medications of this type. In addition, St. John's wort may conceivably interfere with the action of the antitumor drugs etoposide (VePesid), teniposide (Vumon), mitoxantrone (Novantrone), and doxorubicin (Adriamycin).

As for most herbs and drugs, St. John's wort's safety in children and pregnant or nursing mothers, and those with liver or kidney disease has not been established.

Other Natural Treatments for Depression

If St. John's wort does not help you, there are other natural treatments you may wish to try. These are described in Chapter 9. Although none has the same level of solid evidence behind it as St. John's wort, all have shown some promise. Please see chapter 9 for safety issues regarding these substances.

Ginkgo and **phosphatidylserine** may be helpful for depression in those over 50. The typical dose of ginkgo is 40 mg 3 times daily of a 50:1 extract standardized to contain 24% ginkgo flavonoid glycosides and 6% terpene lactones. A typical dose of phosphatidylserine is 100 mg 3 times daily.

DL-phenylalanine may also be helpful for depression, taken at a dose of 75 to 200 mg twice daily. The supplement 5-HTP taken at a dose of 100 to 200 mg 3 times daily has also shown promise for depression. Preliminary evidence suggests that S-adenosylmethionine might be a rapid acting antidepressant, but it is so expensive that it is scarcely practical. When depression is accompanied by anxiety, the herb **kava** may be helpful. A typical daily dose should supply 20 to 70 mg 3 times daily of kavalactones.

When depression is accompanied by anxiety, the herb **valerian** may be helpful. A typical dose is 1 to 2 g of dried root, or 150 to 300 mg of valerian extract standardized to 0.8% valeric acid, 20 minutes before bedtime. Valerian may take many weeks of use to achieve full effects.

You can also consider using conventional medications. Many of the modern antidepressants work very well, and although they cause a greater incidence of side effects on average than St. John's wort, many people take them without problems.

And don't forget psychotherapy. It can be highly effective for mild to moderate depression, and if it works it "belongs" to you. Although it's a natural substance, St. John's wort is similar to conventional drugs in that it only relieves the symptoms of depression. Successful psychotherapy may go deeper.

Notes

Chapter One

1. Schulz V, et al. Rational phytotherapy. New York: Springer-Verlag, 1998.

Chapter Two

1. Hubner WD, et al. Hypericum treatment of mild depressions with somatic symptoms. *Journal of Geriatric Psychiatry and Neurology* 7(Suppl. 1): S12–14, 1994.

Chapter Four

1. Balon R, et al. Sexual dysfunction during antidepressant treatment. *Journal of Clinical Psychiatry* 54: 209–212, 1993.

2. Greenberg RP, et al. A meta-analysis of fluoxetine outcome in the treatment of depression. *Journal of Nervous and Mental Diseases* 182(10): 547–551, 1994.

Chapter Five

1. Linde K, et al. St. John's wort for depression: An overview and meta-analysis of randomised clinical trials. *British Medical Journal* 313: 253–258, 1996.

2. American Medical Association. *Drug Evaluation Subscription* 1: 1–13, 1990.

3. Hansgen KD, et al. Multicenter double-blind study examining the antidepressant effectiveness of the hypericum extract LI 160. *Journal of Geriatric Psychiatry and Neurology* 7(Suppl. 1): S15–18, 1994.

4. Hansgen KD, et al. Antidepressive Wirksamkeit eines hochdosierten Hypericum-Extraktes. *Munch. Med. Wschr.* 138: 35–39, 1996.

5. Harrer G, et al. Placebo-controlled double-blind study examining the effectiveness of an hypericum preparation in 105 mildly depressed patients. *Journal of Geriatric Psychiatry and Neurology* 7(Suppl. 1): S9–11, 1994.

6. Reh C, et al. Hypericum—Extrakt bel Depressionen—eine wirksame. *Alternative Therapiewoche* 42: 1576–1581, 1992.

7. Harrer G, et al. "Alternative" Depressionsbehandlung mit einem Hypericum-Extrakt. *Therapiewoche Neurologie Psychiatre* 5: S710–716, 1991.

8. Laakman G, et al. St. John's wort in mild to moderate depression: The relevance of hyperforin for the clinical efficacy. *Pharmacopsychiatry* 31(Suppl): 54–59, 1998.

9. Ernst E. St. John's wort, an anti-depressant? A systematic, criteria-based review. *Phytomedicine* 2(1): 67–71, 1995.

10. Linde K, et al., 1996.

11. Smet P and Nolen W. St. John's wort as an anti-depressant. *British Medical Journal* 3: 241–242, 1996.

12. Physician's desk reference. Montvale, N.J.: Medical Economics Company, Inc., 1997: 938.

13. Suzuki O, et al. Inhibition of monamine oxidase by hypericin. *Planta Medica* 50: 272–274, 1984.

14. Bladt S, et al. Inhibition of MAO by fractions and constituents of hypericum extract. *Journal of Geriatric Psychiatry and Neurology* 7(Suppl. 1): S57–59, 1994.

15. Muller WEG, et al. Effects of hypericum extract on the expression of serotonin receptors. *Journal of Geriatric Psychiatry and Neurology* 7(Suppl. 1): S63–64, 1994.

16. Winterhoff H, et al. Pharmacological screening of hypericum perforatum L. in animals. *Nervenheilkunde* 12: 341–345, 1993.

17. Muller WEG, et al., 1994.

18. Brown D., ed. Quarterly review of natural medicine. Seattle, WA: NPRC, Inc., Summer 1998: 109–111.

Chapter Six

1. Schulz V, et al. Rational phytotherapy. New York: Springer-Verlag, 1998.

2. Weiss RF. Herbal medicine, translated by AR Meuss. England: Beaconsfield Publishers, 1988: 295–297.

3. Kreitsch K, et al. Prevalence, presenting symptoms, and psychological characteristics of individuals experiencing a diet-related mood disturbance. *Behavior Therapy* 19: 593–604, 1988.

Chapter Seven

1. Katon W. The epidemiology of depression in medical care. *International Journal of Psychiatry in Medicine* 17: 93–112, 1987.

2. Broadhead WE, et al. Depression, disability days, and days lost from work in a prospective epidemiologic survey. *Journal of the American Medical Association* 264: 2524–2528, 1990.

3. Wells KB, et al. The functioning and well-being of depressed patients: Results from the medical outcomes study. *Journal of American Medical Association* 262: 914–919, 1989.

4. Physician's desk reference. Montvale, N.J.: Medical Economics Company, Inc., 1997: 938.

5. Woelk H, et al. Benefits and risks of the hypericum extract LI 160: Drug monitoring study with 3,250 patients. *Journal of Geriatric Psychiatry and Neurology* 7(Suppl. 1): S34–38, 1994.

6. Linde K, et al. St. John's wort for depression: An overview and meta-analysis of randomised clinical trials. *British Medical Journal* 313: 253–258, 1996.

7. Linde K, et al., 1996.

8. Smet P and Nolen W. St. John's wort as an anti-depressant. *British Medical Journal* 3: 241–242, 1996.

9. Schulz V, et al. Rational phytotherapy. New York: Springer-Verlag, 1998.

10. Seigers CP, et al. Phototoxicity caused by hypericum. *Nervenheilkunde* 12: 320–322, 1993.

11. Brockmoller J, et al. Hypericin and Pseudohypericin: Pharmacokinetics and effects on photosensitivity in humans. Pharmacopsychiatry (Suppl 2) 30: 94–101, 1997.

12. Linde K, et al., 1996.

13. Smet P and Nolen W., 1996.

14. Baker RK, et al. Inhibition of human DNA topoisomerase IIalpha by the naphthodianthrone, hypericin. *Proceedings of American Association for Cancer Research* 39: 422, 1998.

15. Nebel A, et al. Potential metabolic interaction between theophylline and St. John's wort. Submitted to Annals of Pharmacotherapy, 1998.

16. Baker RK, et al. Catalytic inhibition of human DNA topoisomerase IIalpha by hypericin, a naphthodianthone from St. John's wort (*Hypericum perforatum*). Manuscript in preparation.

Chapter Eight

1. Vorbach EV, et al. Effectiveness and tolerance of the hypericum extract LI 160 in comparison with imipramine: Randomized double-blind study with 135 outpatients. *Journal of Geriatric Psychiatry and Neurology* 7(Suppl. 1): S19–23, 1994.

2. Thase M, et al. A placebo-controlled, randomized clinical trial comparing sertraline and imipramine for treatment of dysthmia, *Archives of General Psychiatry* 53(9): 777–784, 1996.

3. Harrer G, et al. Effectiveness and tolerance of the hypericum extract LI 160 compared to maprotiline: A multicenter double-blind study. *Journal of Geriatric Psychiatry and Neurology* 7(Suppl. 1): S24–28, 1994.

4. Smet P and Nolen W. St. John's wort as an anti-depressant. *British Medical Journal* 3: 241–242, 1996.

5. Vorbach EV, et al. Efficacy and tolerability of St. John's wort extract LI 160 versus imipramine in patients with severe depressive episodes according to ICD-10. *Pharmacopsychiatry* 30(Suppl. 2): 81–85, 1997.

6. Dunlop SR, et al. Pattern analysis shows beneficial effect of fluoxetine treatment in mild depression. *Psychopharmacology Bulletin* 26: 173–180, 1990.

7. Harrer G, et al., 1994.

8. Thase M, et al., 1996.

9. Stewart JW, et al. Treatment outcome validation of DSM-II depressive subtypes. *Archives of General Psychiatry* 42: 1148–1153, 1985.

10. Linde K, et al. St. John's wort for depression: An overview and meta-analysis of randomised clinical trials. *British Medical Journal* 313: 253–258, 1996.

11. Weiss RF, *Herbal Medicine,* edited by A.R Meuss. England: Beaconsfield Publishers Ltd., 1988: 228.

12. Woelk H, et al. Benefits and risks of the hypericum extract LI 160: Drug monitoring study with 3,250 patients. *Journal of Geriatric Psychiatry and Neurology* 7(Suppl. 1): S34–38, 1994.

13. Linde K, et al., 1996.

14. Balon R, et al. Sexual dysfunction during antidepressant treatment. *Journal of Clinical Psychiatry* 54: 209–212, 1993.

15. Linden J, et al. Fluoxetin in der Anwendung durch niedergelassene Nervenarzte. *Munch Med Wschr* 134: 836–840, 1992.

16. Stokes PE Fluoxetine: A five-year review. *Clinical Therapeutics* 15(2): 216–243, 1993.

17. Stokes PE, 1993.

18. Vorbach EV, et al. Efficacy and tolerability of St. John's wort extract. 1997.

19. Thase M, et al., 1996.

20. Harrer G, et al., 1994; Vorbach EV, et al., 1997.

Chapter Nine

1. Murray M. The healing power of herbs: the enlightened person's guide to the wonders of medicinal plants. Rocklin: Prima Publishing, 1995: 145.

2. Eckmann F. Cerebral insufficiency treatment with *Ginkgo-biloba* extract: Time of onset of effect in a double-blind study with 60 inpatients. *Fortschritteder Medizin* 108: 557–560, 1990.

3. Schubert H, et al. Depressive episode primarily unresponsive to therapy in elderly patients: Efficacy of *Ginkgo-biloba* (Egb 761) in combination with antidepressants. *Geriatr Forsch* 3: 45–53, 1993.

4. Huguet F, et al. Decreased cerebral 5-HT receptors during aging: Reversal by *Ginkgo-biloba* extract (Egb 761). *Journal of Pharmacy and Pharmacology* 46: 316–318, 1994.

5. De Feudis FV. *Ginkgo biloba* extract (Egb 761): Pharmacological Activitie and Clinical applications: Elsevier: Paris. 143–146, 1991.

6. Heller B. Pharmacological and clinical effects of D-phenylalanine in depression and Parkinson's disease. In *Noncatecholic Phenylethylamines, Part 1*, edited by Mosnaim and Wolf. New York: Marcel Dekker, 397–417, 1978.

7. Beckmann H, et al. DL-phenylalanine versus imipramine: A double-blind controlled study. *Archiv Psychiatrie Nervenkrankheiten* 227: 49–58, 1979. See also Beckmann, H. Phenylalanine in affective disorders. *Advances in Biology and Psychiatry* 10: 137–147, 1983.

8. Poldinger, et al. 1991. 24:53–81.

9. Cenachi T, et al. Cognitive decline in the elderly: A double-blind, placebo-controlled multicenter study on efficacy of phosphatidyl serine administration. *Aging* 5: 123–33, 1993.

10. Cenachi T, et al., 1993

11. Maggioni M, et al. Effects of phosphatidylserine therapy in geriatric patients with depressive disorders. *Acta Psychiatrica Scandinavica* 81: 265–270, 1990.

12. Werbach M. Nutritional influences on mental illness. Tarzana, CA: Third Line Press, 1991: 255–271.

13. Schulz V, et al. Rational phytotherapy. New York: Springer-Verlag, 1998.

14. Munte TF, et al. Effects of oxazepam and an extract of kava roots (piper methysticum) on event-related potentials in a word recognition task. *Neuropsychobiology* 27: 46–53, 1993.

15. Mathews JD, et al. Effects of the heavy usage of kava on physical health: Summary of a pilot survey in an Aboriginal community. *Medical Journal of Australia* 148: 548–55, 1988.

16. Schulz V, et al., 1998.

Index

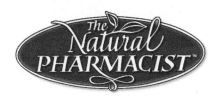

About the Series Editors

Steven Bratman, M.D., medical director of Prima Health, has many years of experience in the alternative medicine field. A graduate of the University of California at Davis, Medical School, he has also trained in herbology, nutrition, Chinese medicine, and other alternative therapies, and has worked closely with a wide variety of alternative practitioners. He is the author of *The Natural Pharmacist: Your Complete Guide to Herbs* (Prima), *The Natural Pharmacist: Your Complete Guide to Illnesses and Their Natural Remedies* (Prima), *The Alternative Medicine Ratings Guide* (Prima), and *The Alternative Medicine Sourcebook* (Lowell House).

David J. Kroll, Ph.D., is a professor of pharmacology and toxicology at the University of Colorado School of Pharmacy and a consultant for pharmacists, physicians, and alternative practitioners on the indications and cautions for herbal medicine use. A graduate of both the University of Florida and the Philadelphia College of Pharmacy and Science, Dr. Kroll has lectured widely and has published articles in a number of medical journals, abstracts, and newsletters.